# SELF-CARE FOR OPTIMUM HEALTH

## Managing Hypoglycemia, High Blood Pressure & High Cholesterol

### Dr. Elvis Ali, ND

# DISCLAIMER

The information in this book are at all times restricted to education, teaching and training on the subject of natural health matters intended for general natural health wellbeing and do not involve the diagnosing, prognosticating, treatment, or prescribing of remedies for the treatment of any disease, or any licensed or controlled act which may constitute the practice of medicine.

Questions? Please email us at: drelvisali10@hotmail.com

# CONTENTS

# ACKNOWLEDGMENTS

It is a pleasure to acknowledge with thanks:

My entire family in Canada and Trinidad and Tobago who have continued to support and motivate me to educate others about naturopathic medicine. My parents, Hakim, Hazrah, my sisters, Alima, Homaida, Homeeda, Fazida, my children, Hassan, Azeeda, Kareem, nephews, nieces and precious grandchildren, Gursimran, Meheirveer and Shairveer for their encouragement and belief in holistic medicine.

Colleagues in the health care profession, especially Dr. Leo Roy.

My students and staff at CCNM, BINM, CCHH, OAND, CAND and clinics, BTNL, AA Comfort Health Centers and Mississauga clinic. The companies for their assistance in educating the public about preventative medicine, Biorrific, Ecoideas, Canadian Bio, Sangsters, Fion Beauty Supplies Canada, Alpha Science Laboratories – A division of Omega Alpha Pharmaceuticals Inc.

My dear friends, Bonita, Pat, Roy, Cindy and Darryl, Janak, Joan, Ash and Harry, Saira and Moe Sheikh of Etobicoke Motors, along with many others too numerous to list.

My publisher and editor Sherree and Lillian who designed the book cover.

# INTRODUCTION

Three of the most prevalent conditions facing millions of people in North America are also the most misunderstood.

I've written this book to dispel some of the myths surrounding hypoglycemia, hypertension and high cholesterol. In most cases, these conditions can be avoided or managed with great self-care. I don't want to call them diseases, because they really are not, as we are led to believe. Yes, they create dis-ease in our bodies, but it is through these discomforts, we are called upon to make better decisions about our eating habits and lifestyle choices.

It's unfortunate that the 'conveniences' of the food industries: fast foods, preserved and packaged foods have contributed to the onset of these ailments. On top of that, the conveniences of technology: computers, telephone gadgets and TV video games are making us more sedentary than ever before. Lack of exercise and just getting out and spending time in nature are also contributing factors.

In my practice as a Naturopathic Doctor, I am often asked: "What do I take to stay healthy?" I will often say that there is no one magic pill since our bodies are so complex and made up of several macro and micro nutrients. Whenever my patients' bodies are out of balance with an illness of some sort, it really means that their whole wellbeing is out of balance: emotional and mental demands, way too much stress and lack of down time, and enjoyment.

As you read through these pages, you will understand that the conditions of hypoglycemia, which eventually leads to diabetes and hypertension (high blood pressure), are usually caused by the wrong types of foods, irregular eating patterns and stress that overload the body's systems and organs. High cholesterol, which eventual cause heart disease and other serious issues, is usually prevented by incorporating the right kinds of fats and oils in our diets.

A commitment to complete self-care can heal these conditions, but there is no going back to once was – the diets and lifestyles that brought them. Your resolve to change is absolutely crucial.

# Hypoglycemia Care

*SUGAR is the fuel of the life of our cells. Every cell and organ of our body needs it.*

*Body energy and heat is derived from sugar. Sugars are the fuels that our muscles need in order to function and work. Our brains use as much sugar in a day as does the rest of the whole body. No cell in the body can function healthily or tolerate deprivation of sugar supplies.*

*HYPOGLYCEMIA is not a disease. It is a word made from three Latin words: "Hypo, means low; "Glyc" means sugar; "emia" (in the) blood.*

*It is an imbalance between the amounts of sugar in the blood and the levels of insulin, due to a breakdown of normal processes of blood sugar regulation.*

*When it is low, every organ of our body is affected.*

## A Story of Hypoglycemia

Most hypoglycemia starts with your breakfasts. Maybe they are rushed. Maybe you are tense or under pressure. Maybe your liver hasn't finished repairing all the wear and tear of your activities and excesses of the day before; it turns the appetite off until its work is completed.

Whatever your reasons or condition, you go for something you call breakfast. A cup of black coffee?  Coffee with sugar? Maybe some milk? Maybe you prefer a big glass of orange juice containing juices and sugars equivalent to eating 3-4-5 oranges? Maybe you take only fruits for breakfast?

Is your breakfast a piece of toast, or a bagel or bun alone; or with the coffee? Do you add some jam or marmalade on your toast? Is it a bowl of dry boxed cereal? Has sugar been added to this cereal? Or you add your own? There is a common denominator in these choices.

They are all sugar foods. There are no foods to balance the sugars as they go into our blood stream. The more sugars or sugar foods you eat, the more sugar goes into the blood. The more these sugars are in a pure form – as in juices or fast digesting foods, the faster they enter into your blood.

All the foods mentioned above fit into this category.
Maybe you don't think you eat much sugar. Maybe a list of foods with their sugar contents will surprise you. Everyone with hypoglycemia needs such awareness.

This list shows approximate amounts of refined and granulated sugar added to and hidden in  popular foods, in addition to their natural sugar content...

| FOOD ITEM | SIZE PORTION | APPROX. SUGAR CONTENT IN TEASPOONFULL |
|---|---|---|
| Orange juice | 6oz | 3 |
| Maple Syrup | 1 Tbsp | 5 |
| Honey | 1 Tbsp | 3 |
| Molasses | 1 Tbsp | 3 ½ |
| Corn Syrup | 1 Tbsp | 3 |
| Fruit Salad | ½ Cup | 3 ½ |
| Canned Fruit | 2 halves and syrup | 3 ½ |
| Stewed Fruits | | 2 |
| Fruit Syrups | ½ Cup | 2 ½ |
| | 2 Tbsp | |
| Donuts – plain | 1 | 3 |
| Donuts – glazed | 1 | 6 |
| Oatmeal cookies | 1 | 2 |
| Cola Drinks | 6 oz | 3 ½ |
| Ginger Ale | 6 oz | 5 |
| 7UP | 6 oz | 3 ¼ |
| Root Beer | 6 | 3 |
| High Balls | 6 | 2 ½ |
| Whisky Sour | 3 oz | 1 ½ |
| Sweet Cider | 6 oz | 6 |

| | | |
|---|---|---|
| Chocolate cake plain | 4 oz | 6 |
| Chocolate cake iced | 4 oz | 10 |
| Chocolate icing | 1 Tsp | 5 |
| Chocolate cookies | 2 | 3 |
| Chocolate pudding | ½ cup | 2 |
| Chocolate bars | 1 ½ oz | 2 ½ |
| Chocolate sauce | 1 Tbsp | 3 ½ |
| Fudge | 1 oz | 4 ½ |
| Cheese cake | 4 oz | 2 |
| Chewing gum | 1 stick | ½ |
| Hard candies | 2 oz | 10 |
| Lifesavers | 2 | 1 |
| Ice cream | 3 oz | 3 |
| Ice cream sundae | 7 oz | 7 |
| Milkshake | 10 oz | 5 |
| Sherbets | ½ cup | 9 |
| Jam, jellies | 1 Tbsp | 4-6 |
| Marmalade | 1 Tbsp | 4-6 |
| Peanut brittle | 1 oz | 3 1/2 |
| Pies | 1 slice | 4-10 |
| Cobblers | ½ cup | 3 |
| Berry tarts | 1 cup | 10 |
| French pastries | 4 oz | 5 |

| | | |
|---|---|---|
| Gelatines, Jello | ½ | 4 ½ |
| Custards | ½ cup | 2 |
| Puddings | ½ cup | 2 - 7 |
| Blanc mangos | ½ cup | 5 |

The more sugar that goes into your blood, and the faster it gets there, the more your body mobilizes processes to utilize these sugars. Our bodies can only use so much sugar in a day. The amounts of daily sugar required to satisfy all our body needs is about four ounces. Your muscles and organs require about two ounces of sugar a day. Your brain requires about an equal amount.

More than this under normal living conditions and your body has to activate means of preventing the blood levels from going too high, for this would be like having diabetes. Your body must burn it up by daily activities or store it, or let it escape through your kidneys. Storage is a function of the liver. What the liver cannot store comfortably will be stored in cells which results in increased fat in cells.

Now, understanding the tremendous amounts of sugar we commonly and unknowingly put into bodies, it is most important you understand what happens in the blood stream as you do this. In grasping this clearly you will know how most people bring hypoglycemia upon themselves – and how you may be doing it to yourself.

In laboratory tests, the sugar levels in blood are measured in milligrams (mgs.) One ounce of sugar equals approximately 30 milligrams. The amount of sugar that is normal in the blood is about 100 mgs., for each cubic centimeter of blood. Any excesses of this are normally filtered from the blood, transformed into glycogen and stored in the liver.

The taking in and using of sugar by the cells, is made possible by insulin. Approximately ½ unit of insulin handles each mg of sugar present in the blood at any one moment. Your pancreas normally secretes the amount of insulin needed to handle each day's sugar intake. It is capable of producing much more.

All efforts – physical, emotional or mental – require energy. They all require insulin. Every cell in our body requires constant and generous supplies of sugar, in order to function, just as engines require fuel. Our brains and nerves, mind and emotions require a great deal of sugar. They burn up as much or more sugar as physical efforts of corresponding intensity. Every act that depletes more energy and nutrient/sugar resources than what is replenished, not only lowers the blood sugar levels, but depletes our vital reserves Now, let us assume that you have had a cup of coffee with a teaspoon of sugar, refined sugar absorbs rapidly into the blood. This adds about an extra 30 mgs of sugar to the blood. The blood passes through the pancreas. The sugar in it tells the pancreas: "Give me more insulin" and the pancreas secretes the needed amount.

Add a piece of toast with some jam on it. These will add about another 30 to 40 mgs of sugar – most of it still the fast absorbing type. Now, the pancreas has to secrete twice as much insulin.
If, instead of the toasts you prefer a donut or a bagel, the sugar levels now go up to mgs. – more than the toast. If what you eat for breakfast is only fruits, the amount of sugar intake and the insulin output to handle it would be about the same. The sugars in starch-grain foods and whole fruits absorb more slowly than the refined sugars or juices of the fruits. This influences the sugar-insulin peaks.

Note how the insulin levels continue to correspond to the levels of sugars, regardless of how high the sugars rise.

Now drink a big glass of orange juice. You have added another approximately 80 to 120 mgs of sugar. A bowl of the usual boxed, dry, flaked, shredded, corn, wheat, rice or similar cereals, together with two teaspoons of sugar and one cup of milk, and the sugar amount increases even more, possibly by another 100 mgs. The amount going into your blood can reach 300 or more mgs of sugar, up to 10 times more than what you should be eating for a whole day.

You have exceeded your day's sugar tolerance level all in one dose. The pancreas now has to secrete up to eight to10 times more insulin than it normally does. You are overloading its capacities and starting to deplete its reserves. However, it has an amazing ability of being able to secrete high doses of insulin for many years. You will notice that the sugar levels peak and decrease rapidly while the insulin levels go down slowly.

## This is where the problem of hypoglycemia arises:

Insulin acts almost immediately. The sugar is reduced close to their normal blood levels, rapidly. The body will not tolerate such excesses for any length of time. But insulin is used up and broken down very slowly. The insulin action can last up to 48 hours.

Within 15 to30 minutes after such meals, all sugars you have taken in have left your blood. Your blood still contains excesses of insulin – maybe even large excesses. It continues nonstop to act on every mg. of sugar remaining in your blood. The sugar levels tend to decrease to low or even very low levels.

These tests indicate that hypoglycemia is, in effect, excess insulin. Excess insulin quickly lowers the blood sugar levels in the blood. As these sugar levels drop below amounts your body requires as fuel and energy for the functioning of all organs, until the next meal you are living on whatever sugar reserves still exist. These reserves are poured back into the blood in order to maintain stable levels required for energetic living.

Eventually, which could mean months or years later, the body reserves will go very low or be depleted. Sugars in amounts that your body needs will not be available. As long as there are reserves, your body is in "hypoglycemic state". This state becomes a kind of emergency. Emergencies trigger a secretion of adrenalin. Adrenalin mobilizes all the body defense systems – including sugars. It also mobilizes the liver to supply, for its reserves, sugars that get stored there. After years of the same process being repeated frequently or daily, eventually the abilities and reserves of the liver become depleted.

Excessive amounts of refined foods and sugars upset the other sugar regulating processes. Insulin is not the only agent which acts on and uses up sugars. Enzymes, vitamins, minerals and trace elements are essential for the efficient utilization of sugars. The more sugars we put into our bodies, which are not accompanied by these enzymes, vitamins, minerals and trace minerals, the more these latter also become depleted. When all compensation processes are depleted, you have become a *hypoglycemic*.

Eventually the insulin productions will go down. The pancreas can over-function for only just so many years. You become a diabetic.

Now, vary the types of foods in your breakfasts. Eliminate the refined sugars, juices, fancy quick commercial boxed cereals and coffee. Add proteins. For example:

- ½ grapefruit; 2 natural fertilized eggs (soft boiled),
- a cereal made from several whole grains, including sesame seeds, millet, flax, buckwheat, together with a one-to-two teaspoons of unpasteurized honey.

This sample substantial food intake has been chosen because it would give you well over 100 mg of sugar, when the eggs and cereals would have digested. But the sugars are slow absorbing. The high quality proteins take time to be digested. Only small amounts of sugar are available to enter the blood, at any moment.

Note that there are no sugar peaks. The sugars are the slow absorbing type foods. They can only pass into the blood when they have been released by the digestion processes, from all the other molecules in the complex foods of which they are a part. The oils in those foods also slow down the sugar release process. The digestion of proteins may take up to a couple of hours. But these proteins are still bound to the sugar molecules. Again, it takes some time to free the sugars. These reach their normal saturation levels by having all the sugars they need.

The amounts of insulin stay constantly on a low level. It can take possibly up to four hours for all the sugars to become a part of the blood flow. They get used up but very slowly in handling sugars. Each unit as it completes its handling of a sugar molecule is available for the next sugar molecules that come into the blood. There is no need for the pancreas to keep secreting any excesses of insulin.

By the time the sugar levels start to drop below your normal levels, you are probably ready for your next meal. The body is satisfied. The sugar balance has been established and made firm for the rest of that day. Any possibility of hypoglycemia ceases to exist.

**Hypoglycemia** can be very distressing and there are over 100 symptoms of hypoglycemia.

**The main discomforts which are most common are:**

| | |
|---|---|
| **Sweating** | **Weakness** |
| Exaggerated hunger | Fatigue |
| Palpitations | Accelerated heart rate |
| Cravings for sweets | Underachievement |

Whatever system is weakened, overloaded or deficient, will react to repeated depletions of blood sugar levels and eventually will damage such organ(s).

Of all organs, the brain and nervous system are the most affected by low sugar levels. When the sugars are low, the brain and nerves demands are not met and we experience:

| | |
|---|---|
| **A lack of concentration, lethargy** | **Insomnia** |
| Psychosomatic problems | Fatigue |
| Mental irritability | Confusion |
| Headaches | Anxieties/fears |
| Blurred vision | Nervousness |

| | |
|---|---|
| Interrupted sleep | Trembling |
| Dizziness | Faintness |
| Low initiative | Insecurity |
| Sensitive emotionality | Lethargy |
| Shakiness when hungry | |

Note, that the hypoglycemia symptoms experienced are very similar to, but must not to be confused with:

| **Body toxicity** | **Allergies** |
|---|---|
| Exhaustion | Burn outs |
| Nervous breakdowns | |

Health problems experienced are frequently nearly identical to those caused by these conditions.

Our body's sources of energy are...

**Foods:** sugars, starches, oils, fats and proteins. Sugars supply immediate quick energy. Starches supply less quick more steady energy.

**Protcins:** Excess is broken down in sugars.

**Rest:** Sleep, relaxation, rest breaks, holidays.

**Atomic:** Fission and fusion of cell biochemical.

**Enzymes:** Activity and biochemical reactions.

**The liver** (our laboratory of life) and all its normal functions and biochemical activities (metabolism).

**Sun:** Magnetism, electricity.

Hypoglycemia is depletion of sugar resources. It is caused by: ALL EXCESS – everything that burns up our life forces, vital reserves and energies.

## Lifestyle Excesses

Everything that burns up our life forces, vital reserves and energies. Over-activity, workaholic, habit excess and insomnia.

## Emotional and Mental Excess

Anxieties, worries, fears, hatreds, angers, repressions, exhilarations and exuberances.

## Physical Excesses

Forced and/prolonged exercises/activities.

## Chemicals – Drugs

Pep pills, diet pills, aspirin and cigarettes.

## Stimulating Foods,

Especially caffeine, tea, chocolate, coffee and cola drink

## High acid foods excess of...

Sugars, sweets, desserts, grains, vinegars, cereals; soft drinks

**Sugar intake** described above, especially taken at breakfast, without proteins. Sugars in refined, processed forms; sugar binges and excesses taken quickly.

**Caffeine, Nicotine, Alcohol** also trigger the secretion of insulin excesses.

## High Tyramine Foods:

Tyramine is an amino acid (a protein), which the body uses to create substances which activate body metabolism. They can induce hypoglycemia. These are proteins that have undergone fermentation, such as aged cheeses, yogurt, fermented grains, sauerkraut, etc.

## Vitamins, Minerals

B Complex vitamins, Sodium

Most vitamins are all stimulants. All the refined, processed, chemically treated vitamins are stimulants.

Vitamins, by nature are activators of enzyme systems. – our body's metabolizers and functional agents.

Vitamin B complex plays three major roles on sugar. It stimulates the liver to create more sugar from glycogen, the form in which sugar is stored in the liver. It helps activate the pouring of this sugar into the blood. It increases the utilization of sugar by the body.

## Stresses, Excesses

Tensions, shocks, strains, pain, infections, exams and study, competitions.

## Endocrine Gland Over-activities

Hormones cause the body to burn up sugar reserves and lower their levels in the blood.

## Under-functioning Glands

Sugars that are not used up (metabolized) will accumulate in the blood, activating the production of excess insulin.

**Adrenals:** Secretions of adrenalin – cortisone. Adrenalin is a powerful liver whip. It speeds up the transfer of glycogen into sugar. It speeds up the flow of blood with this sugar, into the body.

**Thyroid:** This gland acts as a body thermostat. When a body requires more heat and energy, its hormones intensify the burning up of body sugar as a fuel for organ needs.

**Male Glands:** Intensify muscle output.

**Female Glands:** Intensify emotional output.

**Pituitary Gland:** Its hormones activate and accelerate the functions of adrenal, thyroid, and male/female hormones. They increase all body-mind-emotion metabolism and sugar needs.

**Liver Exhaustion:** The liver not only manufactures energy through biochemical reactions, but it is the main storage organ of sugar reserves (in the form of glycogen) in the body. Everything that overloads and drains the liver markedly affects and depletes sugar reserves and fosters hypoglycemia.

**Digestive Enzyme Depletion:** If foods are not normally digested and made available for body use, inevitably there will be a privation of blood sugar as well as the other nutrients.

**Protein Depletion:** Proteins stabilize energies made from sugars. They combine with sugars, slow down their entry into the blood stream and the burning up of these sugars in the blood. They prolong the availability of sugars to the whole body.

The constant availability of quality proteins is essential to energetic wellbeing.

**Not enough proteins and oils:** These are slow burning, long lasting fuel foods.

### Suggested Hypoglycemia Regime

First the "Don'ts": **Never...**

- Take large amounts of sugar at any one meal.
- Take more than four ounces of sugar in a day. This is the normal maximum body tolerance level.

- Note that milk, carrot juice, dates, grape juice and other fruit juices are high in sugar. These foods are to be used carefully.
- Overload the stomach or body with huge meals. It is preferable to eat several small meals, rather than one large meal.
- Overcooked foods: cooking destroys the enzymes essential to the utilization of foods and the sugars in the foods. Excess heat denatures and hardens proteins, making them unavailable for body use – much like putting clay into the oven before molding it into pottery. By this you lose the important action of proteins on blood sugars.
- Refined, processed sugars, candies, sweets, desserts, instant foods, fast and junk foods: These artificial, denatured, chemically treated sugars filter too rapidly into the blood stream. Sugar levels rise rapidly. They overload the liver.

The "Dos" for Hypoglycemia Control

**Always...**

- Make sure that there is a quality protein breakfast. There should be a 'quality protein' at every meal.
- Take frequent snacks, especially when experiencing an energy low (hyperinsulinism). Use two-to-three extra small snacks during the day, to offset insulin excesses, to replenish liver reserves the body needs for immediate sugar energy.
- Your snack should preferably be proteins. Nuts are excellent; a teaspoon of pasteurized honey, with ground nuts or peanut butter, as a quick pick-me-up is excellent.
- Restrict concentrated and fast absorbing sugar foods when blood sugar is low. Rice requires 60 percent less insulin, corn and oats, 30 percent less than normal sugars.
- Control, eliminate, correct as much as possible all hypoglycemia causes, listed above. This may require an

evaluation of a multitude of details, such as information about your diet, your lifestyle and excesses, your habits, your emotions, tensions, work-life, playing and activities, the health of your glands, pancreas and liver. From these will emerge patterns described above which flood the blood with sugar, then with insulin.

Current research and awareness that comes with dealing with thousands of "hypoglycemic" patients, indicates that a properly balanced diet is a most effective basis for treating hypoglycemia. Diet management includes complex carbohydrates with adequate (not excessive) protein.

Diet of frequent small meals, rich in complex carbohydrates and dietary fiber will help maintain a stable blood sugar level.

Timing of meals and snacks can be critical in controlling blood sugar levels. Plan to eat at four-to-five hour intervals. Even prepare meals and snacks in advance and carry them with you.

The conversion of protein and fat containing foods into blood sugar occurs at a slower rate than carbohydrate foods and does not stimulate a rapid flow of insulin.

Sugar levels are controlled by endocrine glands: the pituitary, adrenals, thyroid, pancreas and gonads, as described above.

Hypoglycemia may not be a disease or necessarily a serious condition, but it is often a complex state. It may be simple in the beginning. Don't keep teasing your body with all the conditions that can cause hypoglycemic conditions for too long. The cost to your health may be higher than you want to pay.

## Why refined sugar ruins your health: 69 reasons

**Note:** The following apply predominantly to the unnatural, refined, processed, or chemically created sugars:  the white granulated sugars, glucose, fructose, brown sugar, corn syrup and foods that contain them.

Sugar taken in the form of fruits, fruit juices, starches, honey, molasses and maple syrup, create similar hazards, but only when taken in large excesses.

The sugar substitutes (aspartame, Sweeta, sucryl, saccharine), the sweeteners in diet drinks and diet foods, do not create the same problems, because they are pure chemicals, they are drugs and the problems they can cause may be even worse.

## Sugar Excesses...

1. Cause of hypoglycemia.
2. Elevate blood glucose and insulin in users of oral contraceptives.
3. A major cause of diabetes.
4. Over-activate enzymes and deplete enzyme reserves.
5. Create a strong acid irritating to the stomach (sugars are very acidic).
6. Cause changes which lead to stomach and/or duodenal ulcers.
7. Block absorption of nutrients into the body.
8. Irritate the walls of intestines and bowels and help cause bowel disease.
9. Increase the risk of Crohn's disease and Ulcerative Colitis.
10. A major cause of intestinal (toxic) gas.
11. Can interfere with the absorption of proteins.
12. Can reduce (valuable) high density lipoproteins.
13. Can increase elevation of hazardous low density proteins.
14. Can help denature structures and values of proteins.
15. Raise fasting blood levels of glucose and insulin.
16. Condition the body to alcohol addiction.
17. Help suppress the immune system.
18. Can add to the risks of free radicals in the blood.
19. Causes damage which fosters and promotes aging.
20. Help aging in the skin by denaturing the skin collagen.
21. Induce the adrenals to secrete too much adrenaline into our blood stream ( more so in children)
22. Upset the minerals (mineral balances) in the body.
23. Cause deficiency of copper. (Copper is the nucleus of the enzyme which is the core of Vitamin C).
24. Interfere with the absorption of calcium and magnesium.
25. Induce food form chromium deficiency.

26. Promote an excess of neurotransmitters (serotonin) to saturate the blood.
27. Strongly irritate the nerves and nervous system.
28. Cause insomnia.
29. A major cause of fatigue, (Chronic Fatigue Syndrome, Epstein Barr's Syndrome).
30. Causes agitated restless sleep, dreams and nightmares.
31. Produce a significant rise in triglycerides.
32. Weaken our defenses against bacterial infections.
33. Seriously overload and weaken the liver; in doing so, they add to the possibilities and onset of...
34. Hemorrhoids
35. Varicose Veins
36. Help promote the formation of gallstones.
37. Deplete liver reserves of healing powers.
38. Create conditions favoring formation of kidney stones.
39. Help cause kidney damage.
40. Contributes to the onset of emphysema.
41. Help weaken eyesight.
42. Help cause cataracts.
43. A contributing cause of cancer of the breast, ovaries, intestines, prostate and rectum.
44. Contribute to and foster arthritis.
45. Contribute to and foster asthma.
46. Cultivate conditions that foster growth of Candida Albicans (yeast infections).
47. Is a contributing cause to heart disease.
48. Is a contributing cause to blood vessel disease – hardening of the arteries.
49. Irritate appendix – helps bring on appendicitis.
50. Help reduce resistance to Multiple Sclerosis.
51. A major cause of tooth decay.
52. A major cause of periodontal disease (gums).
53. Can contribute to and favor osteoporosis.
54. Can decrease sensitivity to insulin.
55. Decrease glucose tolerance.

56. Create conditions causing allergies – together with their side effects (especially in children).
57. Drowsiness.
58. Hyperactivity, or
59. Decreased activity.
60. Anxiety.
61. Difficulties concentrating.
62. Irritability and crankiness.
63. Migraine headaches.
64. Can hinder functions of growth hormones.
65. A contributing factor to increased cholesterol.
66. Add to the causes of toxemia during pregnancy.
67. Irritate skin, and act as another cause of eczema – especially in children.
68. Can damage structures of DNA(Chromosomes).
69. Contribute greatly to obesity.

# Blood Pressure Care

*It is not your blood pressure that needs caring for...*
*The pressure of your blood is caring for you;*
*It is the causes of your blood pressure that need your*
*attention and care!*

*As one of the most common conditions and hazards of our civilization, while living in our civilization, understanding its nature and causes becomes most important.*

*Is high blood pressure inevitably a doom?*
*Or is it possibly a boon?*

Blood pressure starts with the vigor with which the heart impels the blood flow through your blood vessels.

High and low blood pressures are recognized by the use of an instrument, which measures the end result of that battle. When the blood is forced through the arteries at a pressure higher than 140 mm. of mercury, it is considered to be high. Above 160 mm. of mercury indicates serious problems or disease exist.

Blood pressure becomes a condition to deal with when it develops into a battle between the power of the heart and any resistance to the flow of blood against this heart power. The object of the battle is always to keep blood flowing with enough force so that this blood can reach every cell in the body and supply them with the nutrients and oxygen they need from normal and vigorous living, then carry off from those cells all the waste products of their functioning.

If your heart pump is tired or lacking in some of its nutrient needs, the pressure goes down. If the heart is overworked and pushes your blood through your arteries with a pressure higher than 200-220 mm mercury, or if the blood is hindered in its return to the heart and accumulates in amounts greater than the arteries or veins can cope with, your blood pressure rises.

Excess high blood pressure is a threat to the thin walled capillaries of the brain. Excess blood stretches the blood vessel walls beyond their elasticity. This can rupture or tear a hole in a vessel wall and allow blood to escape into the brain. This hemorrhage, even if minute, is a stroke.

Blood pressures are always the result of the heart's abilities to keep the blood flowing according to all body needs, and against all abnormalities and conditions which hamper or tend to block this flow.

Our bodies do not make mistakes. In our natures there is a miraculous wisdom and power that governs, with unbelievable accuracy and perfection, everything that exists in our bodies or happens to them.

Every activity, every function, every reaction (even those which seem to be wrong and abnormal activities, functions or reactions) is an ingenious physiological process devised, by its innate wisdom, to handle every body's need and problem in the most perfect way possible, according to the circumstances and conditions in which the body finds itself.

Changes of blood pressure, as they adapt to a body's needs or problems, are not body mistakes. The mistakes are the abuses, demands, excesses, or negligence that we allow into our lives and bring upon our bodies. To compensate for them, the body needs more.

To better and more easily understand blood pressure, its care, and the explanations in the pages that follow, it would most helpful if you would make a picture in your mind and see the blood circulation as being a plumbing system. Visualize your blood circulation as an engineer would. The arteries and veins are like a closed circuit of pipes through which flow fluids propelled by a pump.

When problems arise, like a faulty pump, or a pump pumping to excess, too fast or out of control or there are problems in the pipes (buildups of sediment, blockages, or a narrowing), the body compensates for and overcomes them by pumping blood at an increased pressure.

When any one or more of such problems exist, the fluids accumulate and fill the pipes. As more water is forced into the closed circuit, the excess volume increases the pressure existing in those pipes.

Now back to you and your blood circulation. Central to these circuits is a pump – your heart. Your heart has two chambers, which contract and expand like pistons or pumps. One chamber projects a flow of blood into the lungs. Here the blood saturates itself with oxygen that it will carry to every corner of the body. The other chamber pumps the blood into...

- The stomach, pancreas and intestines, so that they can process ingested foods and prepare them for body use.
- The kidneys. Water that makes up the blood and water soluble impurities is filtered and eliminated.
- The head, whole body, limbs, muscles, bones, skin and every organ, and tissue of the body.
- The liver, where all the nutrients are transformed into molecules acceptable and usable by cells and all your cell wastes, and debris are processed, detoxified, neutralized and eliminated.

Whatever blood gets pumped into your blood vessels must, obviously, come out of your veins, or else, as more blood arrives the volume of fluids will increase. They will create a pressure on your blood vessel walls.

Blood is the lifeline of our lives. Provisions of substantial flows of blood to every organ and cell must be maintained above all other need. Your heart works to provide blood, nutrients and oxygen to maintain health, and perfection.

## Low Blood Pressure

Whenever any health problem exists, extra blood is always required to bring to the needy area or organ more blood, oxygen and nutrients for healing. If your heart is not pumping enough blood to keep your body completely nourished, your energies and vigor high, and every organ functioning at its optimum, it is not to be disregarded or neglected.

If there is no increase in flow of blood to help correct a body need, if there is no rise of blood pressure, if the body fails to respond to a call to arms, if the body is unable to marshal extra defenses to offset abnormalities or changes, or to fight, which are undermining your state of wellbeing then, obviously, you do have a problem. Illness will eventually, inevitably, occur. There is as much reason for concern as when there is any other imbalance, deficiency or toxicity.

A state of lowered levels of life force may not be a disease in medical language, but it is an abnormality that is a reality. You may not need a drug, but you certainly need to take a serious look at everything that provides or maintains your body's vital forces.

Low blood pressure may indicate one or several of the following...

- The energies of heart and muscle are low – the body is exhausted. Healing abilities are low. Your body is run down and depleted, too debilitated to be able to provide for or compensate for its needs.
- The blood vessels lack the strength and/or elasticity to contract. Instead they are distending.
- Your nerves and nervous system that stimulate metabolism and trigger the release of energies and activate your heart and muscles are under-functioning.
- Biochemicals that normally activate the heart and blood vessels are in deficient supply.
- Hormones of the pituitary, thyroid and adrenal (stress) glands, responsible for activating and sustaining the flow of blood and energies throughout your body, are not being secreted in sufficient amounts. Tired or exhausted by stress, traumas and tensions these glands become underactive.
- Chemicals, drugs or toxic substances are depressing the energies of your heart pumping action. They are depressing or depleting the tone of your blood vessel walls – their normal, healthy state, vigor and tension. They are poisoning your blood vessel tissues and causing them to be too loose and lax, rendering them unable to sustain a pressure that is needed to keep your blood flowing freely.

This could mean and create a need for...

- More life forces in your foods
- More rest, relaxation or sleep
- A decrease in lifestyle excesses, stresses or abuses that deplete your body of its energies.

- A restoration of the organs that create life in the body, mainly your liver.
- A restoration of the organs, which activate and sustain the flow of blood and energies throughout your body: your pituitary, thyroid and adrenal (stress) glands.

## High Blood Pressure

When your blood pressure goes up, your body is trying to help you overcome punishments you have imposed upon it. It is forcing extra amounts of blood to the brain, organs and tissues to offset the stresses or abnormal state you have lived to excess. It is trying to correct, heal or eliminate the abnormalities you have created.

An increase of (high) blood pressure is a 'reaction', a symptom. At no time does the body wisdom increase the pressure by which it pumps blood through your body to levels which are not needed or which would be detrimental, unless you override this wisdom, disregard the laws of nature by which your body must abide, and force your body to do so.

Your body, with ingenuity in its best possible way, is responding to or reacting to the other things that are wrong or abnormal. Body discomforts and symptoms that accompany a high blood pressure are 'red flag' warnings that help us become aware that something is wrong and warns us that a threat to your health exists.

Since few people treat their bodies, minds, emotions and organs with kind and deserving care and attention, high blood pressure is quite common.

We should dispel common beliefs and anxieties that minor increases of blood pressure are 'bad', 'wrong' 'disease'. They are not an incurable 'killer' nor a problem without solutions, or problems beyond the scope of modern science.

The pressure of the blood is not the disease. It doesn't make sense that a normal and essential physiological body function should be diagnosed or considered as a 'disease'. The abnormalities which increase the demand for more blood, or which block and hamper the flow of blood, are the real disease and that which needs to be treated.

Blood pressure is a 'disease' only when it is so high it eventually threatens to excessively stretch, damage or rupture weakened blood vessels and secondarily create serious effects and complications.

## The nature of, and reasons for, an increased blood pressure

An increase of blood pressure does not and cannot happen unless there is a reason for it. There has to exist a need, a health problem. There are eight main reasons for every increase of blood pressure:

1. The body as a whole or some tissue, or organ needs more blood. Your heart is pushing harder to make more blood flow through its vessels. Any and every abnormal condition, disease, problem, overload, or organ damage, will, and must, trigger the body to provide more blood.

2. Your body is trying to protect itself against drugs, poisons, abnormalities, excesses, stresses, abuses, or other health hazards and undermining factors and not succeeding as well as it must.

3. Your body is striving to supply more nutrients and oxygen to heal, to repair, to restore and/or to maintain optimum wellbeing to organs subjected to overloads or to emergency needs.

4. The pressure forcing your blood to circulate is less than back pressures, encumbrances or blockages, created by a stagnating blood in the arteries or veins.

5. The flow of blood through an artery or a main area of the body is being hampered or blocked by a buildup of sediments, or plaque, calcium or cholesterol. More pressure is needed to get the blood past this impediment.

6. The blood vessel walls are no longer elastic as they must be. Blood vessels have contracted or narrowed. The size and capacity of blood vessel inner spaces is decreased. Blood vessels must be able to stretch and expand when

extra amounts of blood flow into them. This expansibility prevents blood pressure build ups.

The elasticity of blood vessels, like other tissues, depends on the quality and number of elastic fibers that permeate the vessel walls and tissues. This in turn depends on your body's ability to create these fibers, which is a function of Vitamin P and its enzymes which are fractions of the Vitamin C complex.

Any loss of elasticity of blood vessels leaves their walls very fragile and vulnerable. Since some of the most fragile blood vessels in your body are in your brain, and if the pressure of the blood increases excessively in the brain, and if one of these should break, some blood will leak into the brain. We call this a stroke. Pressure against nerve centers in the brain hinders or damages their function(s).

7.  The muscles of the walls of these vessels are in a state of excessive or chronic contraction. They can no longer expand and hold a volume of blood as they have been called to do.

8.  The contraction of blood vessel wall muscles is controlled by nerves. Over-stimulated nerves create muscle tenseness, contraction and spasm.

    Any state of pressure lower than what is capable of assuring a complete blood and nutrient flow to your body is felt by nerve endings. It activates nerves.

    Nerves signal to the brain: "I need more blood." The brain computer translates these signals into stimuli that trigger the heart to pump more blood, or to pump blood more forcibly. An increased force or contraction of the heart muscles propels extra supplies of oxygen and nutrients through the blood vessels.

To understand excess blood pressure CAUSES is to understand high blood pressure.

The main and common conditions and/or abnormalities that increase blood pressure are listed below – 25 of them, under six main categories. Each of them is explained further on, in the pages that follow.

## Causes of High Blood Pressure

Obstacles to free blood flow result from...

1. **An overloaded, congested and clogged liver, lungs and /or kidneys, by cell debris, tissue wastes and toxic, dead foods.**
   a. Hardening and/or narrowing of the arteries created by deposits of cholesterol and calcium.
   b. Failure to exercise and utilize the muscle contractions as auxiliary blood flow pumps.
   c. Allergies.
   d. Cigarettes: just a few puffs triggers spasticity narrowing of blood vessels.

2. **Blood that is too dense and thick** like molasses that flows only under pressure...
   a. Excesses of blood alkalinity and alkaline minerals. High blood potassium and calcium.
   b. Thickening of blood consistency by gluten.
   c. Decreased body hydrochloric and phosphoric acid resources. Acids are blood thinners.
   d. Some blood diseases. Leukemia with its great excesses of white blood cells.
   e. Excess fats and cholesterol in the blood.

3. **Stimulants that create tension throughout the body and whip the heart to pump too forcefully, put the nerves and blood vessels into contraction...**
   a. Tensions, worries, anxieties, fears and angers
   b. Overwork, lifestyle overloads
   c. Stresses, traumas, shocks
   d. Excesses of abnormal acids: high acid foods, vinegar, soft drinks, fatigue acids – all these are uncompensated for by alkalizing minerals.
   e. Pep pills and appetite reducing pills

    f.   Pollutants in air, water or foods
    g.  Excesses of activating hormones from the thyroid, pituitary and adrenal glands
    h.  Drugs, including many prescription drugs
    i.   Stagnating colon toxins when constipated
    j.   Salt and sodium excesses

**4. Emotions, complexes and sensitivity...**
    a.  Guilt, excesses of obligations
    b.  Angers, fears and resentments
    c.  Repressions and frustrations
    d.  Complexes relating to birth control pills and IUDs

**5. Loss of blood vessel wall elasticity**, which makes it impossible for blood vessels to accommodate increased volumes of blood from causes above.

**6. Excess thinning of blood...** It is obvious from this list, the problem of high blood pressure can be complex. The body, mind, emotions are always complex. Sometimes only one serious abnormality is acting as cause and responsibility for your problem. Sometimes several causes work together. They create problems just as would one serious cause. It is important to note that most of the causes listed, taken separately, are simple. They are related to our body physiology and how we live and treat our bodies. Such causes do not require radical drug intervention. Nor will taking drugs correct or cure what we do to ourselves.

Health problems that arise from multiple interacting causes cannot be eliminated or controlled by a single drug or any simple, single therapy.

# Mechanisms and processes which buildup blood pressure

## 1. Toxicity and Body Pollution

No one can live in our civilization, environment and with all the chemicals and ecological hazards without being polluted by toxicity. Everything we eat, drink and/or breathe adds to the poisons that infiltrate our bodies.

Body organs (like sponges retaining excesses of garbage), can become overfilled with body wastes. The excesses of wastes and toxins stagnate. They collect in and plug up the spaces between cells of organs. Little or no space remains for incoming blood to flow freely through the tissues. Blood collects in the veins that lead to congestion and dammed up tissues.

Toxins, chemicals, body wastes, allergens, excesses, all abnormalities, irritate and whip nerves that penetrate all blood vessel walls. Whipped nerves cause contractions and spasticity of artery walls. Spasticity increases resistance to blood flow. Heart contractions must become stronger. All these increase the pressure of blood.

Often, blood pressure has nothing to do with the body and its functions, nor with what you are eating. It results from strong negative emotions "that are eating you". The mind plays a major role in all the increase of blood pressure.

The brain being the most important organ of the body, the blood in its wisdom, goes there first. Abnormal emotions, as well as chemicals, trigger signals to the brain. The brain, in turn, sends signals that whip the heart and body metabolism to respond to the situation. More blood is pumped under high blood pressure.

Our body constantly strives to flush out all toxins, poisons, wastes and chemicals that could be hazardous. Toxins are eliminated, via the liver, kidneys, lungs and skin, with the liver handling the greatest load. But, flushing requires more blood than the normal flow.

The organ where most congestion and blockage of the flow of blood increases pressure is the liver.

## 2. Livers become congested when...

Overloaded from excessive eating, lifestyle abuses, chemically treated, denatured, dead foods.

The flow of blood through it becomes slow and sluggish as a result of weakened propulsion of blood through the body when heart muscles lose their strength. Any decrease of the blood flow fails to flush out the liver.

## 3. Kidneys

Overloads of body wastes and poisons that are not processed by the liver are "dumped" onto the kidneys. These add to the load of water-soluble toxins the liver normally filters, handles and eliminates.

When the kidneys become overloaded, they send signals to the brain for help. The brain responds by sending out its own signals through the nerves. The nerves increase the flow of blood to the kidneys. Increases of blood and toxins in the kidneys trigger a special mechanism, which increases blood pressure throughout the body.

## 4. Blood Density and Consistency

The body must, and does, maintain exact blood density and consistency at all times. If your blood should temporarily become too viscose, automatically the blood transfers more fluids into it to dilute and restore it to its normal consistency. But this inflow of fluids creates an increase in volume. If the condition persists for any length of time, there will be an increase of blood pressure.

Cell sledging, blood clotting, excess of blood proteins and alkaline minerals, all increase blood thickening. Thick blood flows through arteries and veins slower and with great difficulty. It is harder to pump. The heart beats harder. The blood pressure increases. Blood alkalinity results from excess breakdown of cells. Excesses of lifestyle and living, and excess fatigue make cells die faster and in greater numbers. Cells are rich in potassium, the most alkaline mineral. Excess dying of cells releases excess potassium into the blood. Potassium thickens the blood and slows its flow.

We cause blood alkalinity and thickening by taking too many and too strong alkalizing substances. Antacids commonly used to neutralize excess acids in the stomach, increase the blood alkaline levels. They hinder normal minerals' solubility and interfere with mineral metabolism. They increase blood pressure.

It is important to consistently avoid excesses of these.

### 5. Abnormally Thick Blood – Glyemia

Glyemia is a technical term meaning, "blood glue". Mixing flour (gluten) with water makes glue. Gluten entering into, and mixing with the blood fluid, thickens it. Blood turns into "glue". Man developed strains of wheat (most Canadian and American types), which contain about five times greater levels of gluten than the normal, original wheat.

Blood thickened by factors mentioned above, passes through small blood vessels and capillaries, only with great difficulty. Accumulation and stagnation of blood in these small vessels and capillaries blocks the general flow of blood - a rise in blood pressure results.

Rye flour breads contain about one-seventh or one-eighth of the gluten found in North American wheat. Use these instead of wheat.

In sprouting, seeds digest and use up all the gluten. Use breads made from sprouted wheat.

### 6. Abnormally Thin Blood

Our body wisdom does not tolerate blood thinning. There is only a seeming contradiction in the fact that high blood pressure can be caused by blood that is too thin, as well as blood that is too thick.

Mechanisms for maintaining stable blood consistency come into action. They stabilize blood thickness by allowing a considerable amount of the blood fluid to filter out and exit through the blood vessel walls. Water exits from blood vessels into surrounding tissues when the blood is too thin, as for example, in anemia and conditions of protein deficiencies.

This fluid will accumulate around the blood vessels, like an edema. The tissues that surround the blood vessels swell up. The tissues swelling create a pressure on the outside of, and surrounding, blood vessel walls. The swelling compresses the blood vessels. Pressure makes it impossible for the blood vessels to dilate and expand, as they must whenever the volume of fluid coming into them is excessive. The result is an increase of blood pressure.

## 7. Arteriosclerosis – Hardening of Arteries

Inadequately solubilized or utilized minerals, excess cholesterol, fats, mucus, dead cells, fungi and bacteria can deposit in blood vessel walls. They thicken in these walls. They block the capillaries which feed the artery walls. They harden the arteries.

Deprived of their nutrients and oxygen, the cells of the artery walls lose their vitality and resilience. The artery walls age and become more brittle. Brittleness, loss of elasticity, resiliency and inability of the blood vessel walls to adapt to increased inflows of blood, mean increases of your blood pressure.

- Atherosclerosis is the hardening and narrowing of arteries caused by the slow buildup of plaque on the inside of artery walls.
- As these plaques are made, amongst others, of cholesterol circulating in the bloodstream, elevated LDL-C concentrations are one of the risk factors contributing to atherosclerosis.
- Arteries consist of three layers. The outer layer, composed mostly of connective tissue, is essential for the nutrient and oxygen supply of the blood and lymph vessels, as well as for their innervation. Moreover, it provides structural containment for the two layers beneath.

- The middle arterial layer is made of elastic smooth muscle cells providing contractile strength (expansion and contraction).
- The inner layer (endothelium) comprises endothelial cells, which have the vital function of forming a barrier to prevent toxic substances in the blood from entering the smooth muscle cells of the middle layer. Moreover, the endothelium has to react to mechanical forces. such as blood pressure. It releases substances into the middle layer that change the tone or firmness of the artery.

Atherosclerosis starts with changes in the endothelial cell function. Such changes can be, on the one hand, a result of aging, because the self-renewal process weakens with age. Some of the endothelial functions slow down, and as a consequence, the endothelial barrier becomes leaky (endothelial dysfunction). On the other hand, risk factors such as high blood pressure, elevated LDL-cholesterol and triglycerides, smoking, obesity and lack of physical activity may contribute to endothelial dysfunction.

As a result of endothelial dysfunction, white blood cells (monocytes, lymphocytes) adhere to the endothelium involving endothelial impairment. This impairment allows blood cells and toxic substances circulating in the bloodstream to pass through the endothelium and enter the sub-endothelial compartment instead of flowing normally.

Lipid substances, such as LDL particles accumulate in this area and become oxidized. As a result of LDL oxidation, endothelial cells alert smooth muscle cells to initiate a "repair" process, which eventually results in an atherosclerotic lesion. Depending on individual risk factors (see above), fat accumulation continues and the atherosclerotic process accelerates. In the presence of accumulated fat, monocytes mature into macrophages which try to digest the fat. Smooth muscle cells which have migrated to the area also change their nature to scavenge fat. The fat-laden macrophages and smooth muscle cells (called "foam cells") induce chronic inflammation. Together with inflammatory immune cells, foam cells form early atherosclerotic modifications, so-called "fatty streaks". Fatty streaks are not clinically significant, but they are precursors of more advanced lesions.

More advanced lesions ("fibrous lesions") are characterized by the accumulation of lipid-rich necrotic debris and smooth muscle cells. Fibrous lesions typically have a "cap", consisting of smooth muscle cells and an extracellular matrix enclosing the lipid-rich "necrotic core". With calcification, ulceration at the luminal surface, and hemorrhage from small vessels growing into the lesion from the media of the blood vessel wall, atherosclerotic plaques can become increasingly complex.

### 8. Plaques can grow sufficiently large to restrict blood flow

This involves an inadequate nutrient and oxygen supply to the tissue. A tissue ischemia will then occur. However, plaque growth does not always lead to obstruction of the arterial lumen, because atherosclerotic arteries can remodel to accommodate the expanding atherosclerotic lesion while maintaining a near normal arterial lumen. Consequently, large atherosclerotic lesions may be clinically silent.

- The most important complication of atherosclerosis is an **acute occlusion due to the formation and transport of a thrombus** (blood clot), resulting in myocardial infarction or stroke.
- The underlying basis for 70 to 80 percent of coronary thrombi is the fissure or rupture of the fibrous cap. When an atherosclerotic plaque ruptures, thrombogenic components of the plaque are exposed to the blood stream, leading to activation of the clotting cascade, and finally to the formation of a thrombus, which may clog an artery.
- If a thrombus dislodges and becomes free-floating, it is called an embolus. It is not only arteries of the heart and brain that may be affected, but also arteries of the intestine, resulting in intestinal infarctions. Moreover, it has been suggested that there may be an association between atherosclerosis and pulmonary embolism which

usually arises from a thrombus originating in the deep venous system of lower extremities.

- Recent research has provided new insights into the molecular mechanisms of atherosclerotic plaque rupture. It has been found that plaques with a large lipid pool and a thin fibrous cap are more prone to rupture than plaques with a thick cap, partly because a thick cap is more resistant to mechanical stress. The most important determinant of plaque stability; however, is the composition of the cap. The preponderance of inflammatory cells and a paucity of smooth muscle cells may lead to plaque rupture.

### 9. Stomach – Pancreas Problems

A decrease of hydrochloric acid and enzymes blocks the digestion and utilization of proteins and creates a deficiency, and a thinning of blood, which leads to an increase of blood pressure. The levels of an enzyme called lipase, which is responsible for the digesting and breaking down and dissolving of fats, are considerably lower in those with high blood pressure.

### 10. Protein Deficiencies

Proteins are the building blocks of all cells – the stabilizers of acid alkaline balance, and of sugar and sugar levels. They are essential. Their levels must be constant. Normal blood proteins are maintained by an adequate diet intake and their complete digestion by the stomach and pancreatic enzymes.

In order to keep up the supplies of proteins to the cells and tissues, when proteins are too low, the body gets the heart to work harder. Proteins give strength to the heart muscles. The heart mobilizes more blood at a higher blood pressure. If heart muscles are not strong, the blood fluids become sluggish. Fluid sluggishness and stagnation make any further flow of blood into tissues more difficult.

The increase of blood pressure forces more proteins to pass

through blood vessel walls into tissues and cells. Cells that do not obtain sufficient proteins tend to degenerate. This includes the cells out of which the blood vessel walls are constructed.

## 11. Hydrochloric (Phosphoric) Acid Deficiencies

These are essential to maintaining solubility and usability of minerals in the bloodstream. Without this acid action, iron is unavailable for building good blood. Iodine is unavailable  for making thyroid hormones. These hormones prevent the blood pressure from being too low. Calcium cannot help calm nerves and prevent the pressure from going too high. Other minerals are similarly affected. Mineral deficiencies and depletion can be the starting point of high blood pressure in many people. Normal acidity decreases viscosity. It maintains a normal blood thinness.

These acids are a major defense against bacteria that invade the blood and the capillaries of the blood vessel walls. Ninety percent of the most harmful bacteria cannot survive in an acid environment. Hydrochloric acid helps create the tissue environment required for enzymes to produce energy. Hydrochloric acid maintains and adds to the life forces created by cells. Normal energy reserves eliminate the need for extra blood. They normalize blood pressure.

## 12. Deficiencies – Tissues Starvation

**Blood Starvation** (anemia) and other deficiencies of essential elements must be compensated for. The body, by a normal reflex, does this by forcing more blood to flow through the arteries thus increasing the amount of oxygen, enzymes, vitamins, minerals and proteins available to cells.

A body's' sugar levels tend to go low when proteins are low, or when its demands for energy are excessive. Low blood sugar reserves will create the same demands for an increase of blood pressure, as conditions already described.

**Hormones** play a major role in the utilization of proteins and of minerals in the cells. Thousands of body chemicals are stabilized and balanced by the various hormones. Hormone deficiencies will also trigger blood pressure increases to compensate.

Vitamin A (+its enzymes) affects almost every aspect of health. Vitamin A deficiency will influence passage of all nutrients and chemicals through membranes of cells, including the passing of nutrients through intestinal walls, elimination of poisons through kidneys and lungs.

**Vitamin C**(+ its enzymes) is considered the universal vitamin. It partakes in the function of adrenals, lungs, nerves, heart and the elasticity, integrity, and health of all blood vessel walls. Vitamin C is destroyed by drugs, chemicals, poisons, toxins, radiation, and excess heat and by contact with oxygen.

**Vitamin B**(+its enzymes) is equally important. Vitamin B is an essential factor to all of the normal functions of liver, pancreas and nerves.

**Calcium** is the mineral required in the greatest amounts by the body: by bones, ligaments, cartilages, nerves, teeth and the structure of all cells. High blood pressure may follow any inadequate utilization of calcium ions.

**Selenium** is a main element of the enzyme complexes, which are part of the Vitamin E team. When selenium and the enzymes made from selenium are lacking, the Vitamin B complex fails to fulfill its normal functions. Vitamin E protects the blood and its components. It prevents the oxygenation and breakdown of oil soluble nutrients and biochemicals essential to health.

**Chromium and Zinc** are essential for the normal function of the pancreas and liver. They affect the body's ability to produce insulin. Zinc is essential to creating and  the function of more enzyme systems than any other trace mineral.

Deficiencies of any of these vitamins and minerals or other elements always create a need for greater and stronger blood flow.

**Pressures/Stresses.** Overwork, frustrations, repressing or suppressing tensions and anxieties; inadequate release of stresses, all affect the blood pressure. They trigger spastic contraction of muscles throughout the whole body and the compressed blood vessels result in high blood pressure.

A simple WORRY can push blood pressure up 20 points. This is normal. Even wondering if the high blood pressure treatment is helping increases body tensions.

**Fears.** Blood pressure *phobia* can be as much a disease as high blood pressure. It increases the blood pressure by many points. It may be more hazardous to health than the moderately high levels of blood pressure.

There are no justifications for fearing blood pressure or stroke until...

- Pressure rises above 200 to 225. Only extremely high blood pressures can damage our bodies. What 'kills' are the *causes* of the blood pressure.
- Arteries are so brittle and fragile that they are like tissue paper.
- The world is clamping down on you with pressures that are intolerable.

### 13. Heart Muscle Weakness and Failure

Any lessening of the force, by which the heart muscles pump the blood through the veins, creates blood stagnation throughout the circulation. Stagnation increases blood pressure. Heart failure can result from most of the problems already discussed..

### 14. Salt Excesses: Tissue Edema

The problem we associate with salt relate only to the common table salt made up of only two minerals: sodium and chloride. These, like all other minerals, must be balanced by other minerals. Sodium must be counterbalanced by potassium. If not, it is a drug. Each ounce of table salt binds and holds one pound of water in the bloodstream and in the body. Excess fluid retentions increase the pressure in the blood.

Sea salt is not detrimental to the body, to blood or blood pressure. It is composed of hundreds of minerals and trace minerals in a formula identical to the mineral formula of blood, and perfectly in balance with the blood, its needs, and the body's needs.

## 15. Adrenal Glands

Adrenal glands create the mechanisms by which our bodies can adapt, even to the greatest of stresses.

However, when adrenal glands are overactive, stresses, tensions, overloads, shocks, trauma, unkind words, strong emotions, stimulate them to overreact. Overactive adrenals secrete excess adrenaline. The adrenaline goes to the heart, forcing it to pump harder and faster, to the lungs forcing them to work harder to provide extra oxygen, and to the liver forcing it to pour more sugar for energy into the blood.

Over-activity of the adrenals, caused by increased blood pressure, can be ascertained by a simple test : the Ragland's Test.

Lie down until completely relaxed. Have your blood pressure taken. Then stand up and quickly take it again. You heart experiences a slight stress as it pumps blood against gravity. Extra blood is required to supply the increased working of muscles. This simple, physical act of standing up boosts up pressure by five points. This is normal.

An increase of more than five points of blood pressure indicates an over-activity of the adrenal glands. If your systolic (the first number) does not rise above four to10 points, suspect hypoadrenia. If your blood pressure drops, you can be sure you have hypoadrenia and you may feel a little faint upon standing.

In my naturopathic practice, I have also known how imperative it is to ascertain the "causes" of "dis-ease" among my patients. Indeed STRESS affects all and it is crucial to address how it plays a part on one's blood pressure. As Dr. Hans Selye mentioned, "It is not stress or stressors that will harm you, rather it is how you perceive stress."

## Stress – Adrenal Exhaustion

In our fast, bustling society today, we have an incredible amount of stresses and our body reacts by mounting a stress response through the stimulation of the sympathetic nervous system. Hans Selye did a lot of research on stress and referred to the "fight or flight" response as the body arms itself to face what it perceives as potential danger. When this happens, epinephrine is secreted from the adrenal medulla, and the hypothalamus-pituitary axis is stimulated to release ACTH, which in turn causes the adrenal cortex to increase production of the anti-stress hormone cortisol.

The adrenal glands, which secrete hormones, are walnut-sized glands, located above the kidney and often become 'exhausted' as a result of the constant demands placed upon them. The outer layer of the gland, called the adrenal cortex, produces hormones including cortisol, DHEA, estrogen and testosterone. The function of the adrenal glands is performed by a wide variety of hormones released by the inner adrenal medulla and the outer adrenal cortex which is mostly directed at the physiological response to stress. The medulla is responsible for producing epinephrine and norepinephrine (adrenaline), which controls the body's reaction to stress and affect blood pressure, heart rate and sweating. The adrenal cortex produces hormones, such as cortisone and aldosterone which are necessary for fluid and electrolyte (salt) balance in the body, as well as regulating the use of dietary protein, fats and carbohydrates and controlling inflammation.

Major health problems can occur when the adrenal glands produce too many or too few hormones. Two disorders caused by impaired functioning of these glands are:

1. Addison's disease. Addison's disease is caused by damage or disease to the adrenal glands, resulting in a deficiency of the hormone cortisol.
2. Cushing's syndrome. The overproduction of cortisol by the adrenal glands leads to Cushing's syndrome.

An individual with adrenal exhaustion will usually suffer from chronic fatigue, may complain of feeling stressed-out or anxious, and will typically have a reduced resistance to allergies and infection. The adrenal glands secrete several important hormones that help maintain the balance of many body functions. Stress, fasting, temperature changes, infections, drugs, and exercise all stimulate the adrenals to release their hormones. When the adrenals release too few or too many hormones, the body responds differently to the everyday stresses of life.

Adrenal fatigue has a broad spectrum of non-specific yet often debilitating symptoms. The onset of this disease is often slow and insidious. When a person experiences chronic stress, the cortisol level may rise to such a high level that its production reduces as the adrenal becomes exhausted.

Under normal conditions, cortisol helps convert proteins into energy, releasing glycogen and counteracting inflammation. For short durations this if fine, but at sustained high levels, cortisol gradually tears your body down. This leads to destruction of healthy muscle and bone; slows down healing and normal cell regeneration; impairs digestion, metabolism and mental function; interferes with healthy endocrine function, and weakens your immune system.

In the early stages of adrenal dysfunction, cortisol levels are too high during the day and continue rising in the evening. This is called "hyperadrenia." In the middle stages, cortisol may rise and fall unevenly as the body struggles to balance itself despite the disruptions of caffeine, carbohydrates and other factors, but levels are not normal and are typically too high at night. In advanced stages, when the adrenals are exhausted from overwork, cortisol will never reach normal levels ("hypoadrenia"). Below lists stressors that can lead to adrenal exhaustion/fatigue.

- Anger
- Chronic fatigue
- Chronic illness
- Chronic infection
- Chronic pain
- Depression
- Excessive exercise
- Fear and guilt
- Gluten intolerance
- Low blood sugar
- Mal-absorption
- Mal-digestion
- Toxic exposure

- Severe or chronic stress
- Surgery
- Late hours
- Anger
- Sleep deprivation
- Excessive sugar in diet
- Excessive caffeine intake from coffee and tea

When the adrenal glands are not functioning optimally, you can have a condition that is known as adrenal fatigue, or adrenal exhaustion. Adrenal fatigue often develops after periods of intense or lengthy physical or emotional stress, when too much stimulation of the glands leaves them unable to meet the body's needs. The following is a list of symptoms that includes:

1. Excessive fatigue and exhaustion
2. Non-refreshing sleep (you get sufficient hours of sleep, but wake fatigued)
3. Overwhelmed by or unable to cope with stressors
4. Feeling rundown or overwhelmed
5. Craving salty and sweet foods
6. You feel most energetic in the evening
7. A feeling of not being restored after a full night's sleep or having sleep disturbances
8. Low stamina, slow to recover from exercise
9. Slow to recover from injury, illness or stress
10. Difficulty concentrating, brain fog
11. Poor digestion
12. Low immune function
13. Food or environmental allergies
14. Premenstrual syndrome or difficulties that develop during menopause
15. Consistent low blood pressure
16. Extreme sensitivity to cold

There are many ways to help with adrenal exhaustion, beginning with a proper medical checkup which includes a physical exam, blood work, saliva testing and/or urine tests. Maintain the following program:

1. Dietary changes to enrich your nutrition and reduce carbohydrates and stimulants. Always have breakfast and smaller meals with snacks.
2. Stress reduction, including moderate exercise (Tai Chi, Yoga or Chi Gong), and taking more time for yourself to relax.
3. Do the things that you enjoy.
4. Get more rest.
5. Avoid coffee or other caffeine containing beverages.
6. Eat early and your last meal should be two hours before bedtime.
7. Have a glass of water(warm) in the morning with ½ squeezed lemon.
8. Avoid grains such as bread.
9. Avoid starchy foods, such as potato and trans fat (fries)
10. Try laughing yoga and avoid getting over-tired.

As with any specific type of treatment, the treatment(s) for adrenal disease should be based on the underlying cause(s). Treatment generally takes the form of synthetic hormones, which increase the low levels in the body, or hormone inhibiting drugs, depending on the disease. Treatment is usually lifelong unless the cause of the disease is removed, such as a tumor which is surgically removed or treated with radiation or chemotherapy.

Due to stressful situations and an unhealthy lifestyle resulting in adrenal damage and fatigue, it is imperative that this situation can be best treated and improved with a holistic and natural approach.

Herbal medicines are well-known for their tonic effect on the adrenal glands and improving ability to cope with stress. Examples include: lemon balm, Foti root, astragalus, green tea, licorice root, Ashwagandha, pomegranate, guarana, borage, Siberian ginseng, borage oil. Combinations of herbs with Aswagandha like Adreanalife can be used to help deal with stress.

Vitamins and minerals are also needed to help cope with stress, especially the B-complex vitamins and Vitamin C. (See table below). Antioxidants are also great to provide more energy and slow the affects from free radical destruction. Some examples are: grapeseed extract, pine bark, alpha lipoic acid, Omega 3,6,9 fatty acids, bioflavonoids, as well as trace minerals, zinc and selenium.

Relaxation methods and reducing stress in one's daily life, as well as eating a healthy, balanced diet and exercising regularly can all be of great benefit to adrenal disease. Here are natural supplements to consider:

| Vitamin | Combine With | Source | Therapeutic Applications |
|---------|--------------|--------|--------------------------|
| B complex | Vitamins C,E, Calcium, phosphorus | brewer's yeast, liver, whole grains | Needed for proper maintenance of the nervous system, proper functioning of the cell and its energy metabolism |
| B1 (Thiamine) | B complex, Vitamins B2, C, E, folic acid, niacin, manganese, sulphur | brewer's yeast, brown rice, fish, meat, nuts, organ meats, poultry, wheat germ | Helps maintain good health. Helps maintain normal growth. Helps the body metabolize carbohydrates. |
| B2 (Riboflavin) | B complex, Vitamins B6, C, niacin, phosphorus | Nuts, organ meats, whole grain | A factor in the maintenance of good health. Helps in tissue formation. Helps the body to metabolize proteins, fats and carbohydrates. |
| B6 (Pyridoxine) | B complex, Vitamins B1, B2, C, pantothenic acid, magnesium, | brewer's yeast, green leafy vegetables, meat, organ meats, | A factor in the maintenance of good health, helps the body to metabolize proteins, fats and carbohydrates, and |

| | potassium, linoleic acid, sodium | wheat germ, whole grains, desiccated liver | helps in tissue formation. |
|---|---|---|---|
| B12 (cobalamin) | B complex, Vitamin B6, C,choline, inositil, potassium, sodium | cheese, fish, milk, milk products, organ meats | Helps in treating pernicious anemia. Promotes heart health. |
| Folic Acid (folacin B complex) | B complex, Vitamins B12, C, biotin, pantothenic acid | brewer's yeast, fish, legumes, organ meats, soybeans, wheat germ, lecithin | Adequate intake helps to maintain good health, produce red blood cells, and helps prevent neural tube defects when taken prior to becoming pregnant and during early pregnancy. |
| Niacin (Niacinamide B complex) | B complex, Vitamins B12, B2, C, phosphorus | brewer's yeast, seafood, lean meats, milk, milk products, poultry, desiccated liver | A factor in the maintenance of good health. Helps normal growth and development. Helps the body to metabolize proteins, fats and carbohydrates. |
| Pantothenic Acid (B complex) | B complex, Vitamins B6, B12, C, biotin, folic acid | brewer's yeast, legumes, organ meats, salmon, wheat | A factor in the maintenance of good health, helps the body to metabolize proteins, fats and carbohydrates, and helps in tissue formation. |

| | | germ, whole grains | |
|---|---|---|---|
| C (ascorbic acid) | all vitamins & minerals, bioflvonoids, calcium, magnesium | citrus fruits, cantaloupe, green peppers | Vitamin C is a factor in the normal development and maintenance of bones, cartilage, teeth and gums, it promotes a healthy immune system and possesses antioxidant activities. |

## Overactive Metabolism – Hyper- (active) Thyroid

The thyroid hormones control and intensify most of your body's metabolism processes. Toxins, be they chemical, mental or emotional, whip the thyroid into a state of over-activity. Overactive thyroid seriously increases blood pressure.

## Allergies

Even minute doses of allergens can act like a toxin or a poison. Allergens in the blood cause the blood vessel walls to contract. They may, even quickly, increase blood pressure by up to 50 points.

A pulse that is fast, a pulse going 18 to 20 beats a minute faster than it should, means that there are toxins or irritants in the blood. Even poorly tolerated foods, to which the body is hypersensitive, can produce such heart accelerations.

Allergens common to many and possible causes of high blood pressure are: milk, coffee, cigarettes, wheat, corn, sugar and alcohol. Many people poorly tolerate the denaturing in pasteurized milk.

Testing routines to determine the tolerability of substances entering into or affecting the body can become a must. Ferreting out allergens may mean the difference between health and disease, between freedom from high blood pressure or suffering its serious complications.

## Stimulants – Irritants

Tea, coffee and cheese are common culprits and strong whips to the nerves and causes of high blood pressure. Decaffeinated coffee can be just as bad, worse than ordinary coffee. Much decaffeinating is done by action of toxic chemicals. Chemicals that replace the caffeine are just as hazardous – or more so.

## Being a Woman

Female extra-sensitivity and emotionality leaves some women more susceptible to tension build ups with resulting increase of blood pressure.

**Pregnancy:** the role of the body in pregnancy is to create a perfect environment for the new baby. Sometimes this overloads and congests the liver. The liver must work extra hard for two bodies.

## High Blood Pressure Care

For generations the medical profession has claim that there is no real cure for high blood pressure. Of course not! How can there be? Blood pressure is not a real "disease". It is not a condition that needs to be "cured". There are times, in blood pressure extremes, that the pressure needs to be strongly controlled or suppressed. However, such controls should be maintained only until the causes can be determined and eliminated.

### *"Cures" consist in eliminating causes – all of the causes.*

*Disorders which trigger high blood pressure are what need to be effectively treated. When, and only when, these are eliminated, you have a cure.*

*Causes will be different for, and specific to, each individual. Regimes and the cures must be tailored to each specific cause – each specific person.*

High blood pressures are generally provoked by multiple

causes – several causes acting in unison together. Multiple causes cannot be eliminated or cured by one single, simple panacea drug or therapy.

There are no simple answers – no panaceas. Basic to each treatment plan is the restoration of all the body's enzymes, vitamins, minerals, proteins and oils required for healing and health maintenance.

Decongesting and detoxifying and maintaining an effective flow of blood through the liver, are a constant and essential part of high blood pressure care. This approach can effectively reduce blood pressure, and it can do this in a relatively short time.

## Controlling Blood Pressure Phobia

Fears are gestated by 'not knowing'. Much of our panic arises from the beliefs indoctrinated into us by medical doctors and by drug companies who promote the sale of blood pressure drugs. Fears of blood pressure can be eradicated by acquiring understandings of the common sense causes and what to do about them.

Early stages of increased blood pressure are not a reason for anxiety or panic. However, it is a "red flag", warning you and your doctor...

- To ferret out the presence of any severe deviations from optimum health
- To find and determine the nature of any hampering or blocking of blood circulation
- To determine how serious are the body's needs for more blood
- How damaging to the body or an organ are the blood pressure increases

If you feel fearful of abandoning blood pressure pills, perhaps you haven't taken a good look at your body, its needs and how it functions and protects itself.

## Drugs and High Blood Pressure

In cases of extremely high blood pressure, the use of controls and drugs may be advised to temporarily – until the nature of the causes can be determined and eliminated. There are some immediate benefits associated with taking of high blood pressure pills. Excesses of blood or body fluids will be eliminated. Drugs will curb the blood pressure from rising excessively. The symptoms and the consequences of high blood pressure will be temporary relieved. Blood vessel accidents and strokes will be delayed. But drugs cannot stave off eventual tragedy.

Drugs always stimulate the adrenal gland. This gland will manufacture cortisone and adrenaline. These always make your body feel better - temporarily.

Drugs can paralyze the nerves and stop their effect on blood vessels and body organs that foster the increase in blood pressure. They could lower the pressure. They can also drug your body into a state of paralysis.

Causes that are allowed to remain active will foster reoccurrence of eventual distress. Extremely high blood pressure can continue to build up in the blood vessels regardless of the number or kinds of drugs taken, as long as the causes which brought on the condition continue to be present and active in a patient. However, at the same time causes will be masked. High blood pressure drugs interfere with one of the body's very important life protecting functions. They block the body's determined efforts to supply your body's needs and maintain health normalness by forcing blood through obstructions in organs or blood vessels.

Drugs do not restore one's original state of a healthy body. Nobody gains health from drugs. Barring extremes, the solution is not to inhibit the body from allowing normal moderate increases of blood pressure. It does not make sense to the body's wisdom to take drugs any longer than to relieve the hazards of blood pressure crises.

Rather than treat blood pressure as the disease, with drugs that do nothing to eliminate the reasons why your pressure is rising, it would seem more reasonable to search out and diagnose the abnormalities that cause the problems, and to determine why the body needs extra blood supplies. These causes are the real disease. These, rather than the blood pressure, are what need to be treated.

**Cures are processes which normalize and eliminate each and all causes.**

To be effective for high blood pressure, a therapy must...

- Treat the person - the whole person, not the symptom
- Provide every element, enzyme, vitamin, mineral, protein and oil needed for total healing, for maintenance of health and for prevention of any recurrence of high blood pressure.
- Include the sound diet of whole, natural, alive foods which are free of additives, pesticides and chemicals (fertilizers) and which have not been denatured by excess cooking.
- Encourage positive and dynamic mental attitudes, allowing normal compromise.
- Control excesses and stresses of lifestyle.
- Balance and control abnormalities of the environment.
- Provide the body with the appropriate balance of both hormones and alkaline and acid minerals.
- Normalize and stabilize the blood density and consistency
- Formulate a program tailored to your specific needs. Control the particular nature, personal individuality, the excesses, lifestyle, stresses and emotional complexes.

**Specific Effective Therapies and Regimes: Detoxification**

Detoxification is an art essential to most cures:

- Detoxify by the use of therapies, laxatives, enemas, dieting, anything capable of ridding the body of every irritant, drug, chemical, excess, body wastes, toxin, and every possible substance unnatural to the body, which the body cannot tolerate.

- Effective intestinal elimination of body wastes by daily use of a combination of high-fiber foods, like oatmeal, bran muffins, can lower a person's blood pressure by up to 10 percent (University of Kentucky research).
- Enhance the activities and deficiencies of the many organs, biochemical systems and functions, whose role is to neutralize, control and eliminate body poisons.
- Detect, determine, eliminate and control all allergens
- Determine and eliminate environmental hazards.

## Detoxify by Fasting

To fast is to give rest to the digestive organs, which allows all energies and enzyme systems of our body to focus on their action to destroy body poisons.

Use generous amounts of liquids. It is a most effective method of clearing out wastes and toxins that will cause high blood pressure or all kinds of other problems in the body.

## Treat Hardening of the Arteries and Cholesterol

- Use lecithin to dissolve cholesterol.
- In severe cases, use chelation a therapy.
- Acidify and solubilize minerals, by the use of hydrochloric acid, and/or phosphoric acids.
- Use trace minerals that increase the metabolism and the potential creation of enzymes.

## Control the Diet

A 'light' diet helps to calm body tensions and blood pressure. Follow a regime predominantly rich in vegetables, fruits, quality oils and proteins.

## Stop foods that whip your system

- Coffee, tea, chocolate, mustard, alcohol and excess acids in the diet. Do not use much sugar or other highly energizing and stimulating foods. Honey energizes, but it does not stimulate.
- Dead foods, junk foods, overcooked and refined foods, commercially processed foods, rich deserts, milk and dairy foods; foods which digest poorly, mucus-producing foods.
- All fats, margarine, hydrogenated oils, chemically treated oils, salad dressings and mayonnaises.
- Meats, fats, cheeses are conducive to increase in blood pressure.

## The Use of Natural Diuretic

Elimination of excess body water is essential. The steady use of mild natural acting diuretics can often provide relief comparable to that provided by diuretic drugs. Some excellent water eliminators are...

- Water – especially distilled water.
- Grapefruit – eating several a day.
- Watermelon – quite an effective remedy.
- Diuretic Teas – silk of corn husks, brewed water. Several herbal teas and tablets for diuretics are sold by herbalists and in many health stores.

## Stress – Excess Controls

For tenseness and excess overloading of organs of the body, such as those which cause high blood pressure, time to rest and relax are specifically needed.

In case of a broken leg, or high fever, or complete exhaustion any physician advises bed rest. Similarly, in cases of constant tenseness and excess overloading of internal organs (two precursors for high blood pressure) the body needs time to rest, relax and recuperate.

Blood pressure pills cannot replace this need.

## Treatments of Liver Congestion

Always, when there is a blood pressure problem, learn to know, understand and care for your liver.

**Exercise** is especially valuable as a frequent practice of deep breathing. Breathing exercises make the diaphragm work like a piston. The diaphragm up and down expansions and contractions work on the liver just as much as it does on the lungs.

At each lung expiration the dome of the diaphragm rises and creates a vacuum below it. This draws the liver up and takes pressure off it and blood from the body flows more freely into the liver. The downward thrust of the diaphragm compresses the liver. This squeezes out blood, as well as excess toxins stagnating in the liver. It decongests.

Stretching helps greatly release tensions. Let muscles and joints tell you what to do (listen to your body) what they need, just like the stomach tells you what your body needs in way of nourishment. Do it whenever and for as long as it feels good. Stretching creates mental release too.

**Liver enzymes** enhance the biochemical detoxifying and flushing out actions and functions of the liver. Some past sources of enzymes are concentrates of beets, milk thistle and dandelion roots.

**Bile** is liquid which dissolves, absorbs, flushes out and carries into the intestines almost all of the breakdown waste products and garbage that congest and block the liver if not disposed of.

## Observations: reactions during therapy

You may expect some reaction when you go off the blood pressure pills, tea, coffee or whatever stimulant is affecting you. People develop hangovers from any kind of drugs, chemicals and body toxins, not just alcohol.

If a treatment has been well followed, it is NOT the blood pressure that causes the migraines. It is the causes, the toxins and pollutants in the body that are highly irritating to nerves, not the blood pressure itself, that can, and often does, cause migraine headaches.

Worrying about the migraine, keeps attention focused on the head, increases circulation to the brain, and adds more tension to causes already present and to blood pressure.

## Learn to listen to your body

Your symptoms and body changes indicate optimum ways to handle health problems. Learn to be sensitive to them, to understand and appreciate them. Your body will respond to feelings of wellbeing when the causes of high blood pressure are eliminated.

We take care of our stomach needs when we are hungry. Why not take care of muscle needs, emotional needs, social needs, nerve needs, energy needs, needs to rest, needs for more enjoyment of living, as our feelings and intuition tell us to do these.

When the body recognizes that normality reigns again, it quietly and quickly turns off the alarm signals as well as the processes that increase pressure building. Health and energy return and exist again.

## The role of a physician is to...

- Treat the emergency of extreme high blood pressure
- Instruct, counsel and guide the patient to complete health
- Avoid pushing pills, be an alarmist or promote hopelessness for this so-called "killer disease" by reinforcing the fear that there is "no effective cure".

# Oils, Fats & Cholesterol Care

According to WHO research, high cholesterol contributes to more than half (56%) of all cases of coronary heart disease worldwide and causes millions of deaths per year.

*Blood pressure can be your friend.*

*Respect it and allow it to help you when it must.*

*Take advantage of the health benefits it can offer*

Every few years the media publicizes a symptom or condition, which until then is considered as of little importance. It is given the label of a new disease. General tiredness becomes Chronic Fatigue Syndrome. Muscle aches and pains become Fibromyalgia. Such announcements generally coincide with the discovery by a drug company of a new drug that offers relief for the new "sickness".

Cholesterol is one of these new style diseases. Doctors, persuaded by drug promotion, inform us that cholesterol causes heart disease and strokes. Well over 600,000 Americans die of these illnesses every year. The drug companies discovered a drug they claim will lower blood cholesterol levels. Thousands of people rushed to their doctors. The doctors run tests. They find abnormal blood cholesterol levels. Cholesterol is now stigmatized as a serious threat to the heart and life. The drug is prescribed. The drug companies rejoice as they watch money roll into their bank accounts.

There is no cholesterol problem. There is no problem related to normal healthy cholesterol. Cholesterol is a normal, essential and important component of the structures and functions of our body. Normal health cannot exist without it. Creating fears and avoiding cholesterol as an evil is not justifiable. Nor is it right to condemn as evils the essential quality oils from which cholesterol is created, or to confuse healthy oils with toxic oils and fats.

This section of the book clarifies the truths and half truths about oils and cholesterol, and the hazards of all fats and to bring to your awareness the differences between healthy and unhealthy cholesterol and between healthy and unhealthy oils.

# Cholesterol

## Cole = bile; ster = hormone-related: ol = oil

**Normal, healthy cholesterol is a nutrient that is absolutely essential for the body and the health, functioning and growth of cells. It is in every cell and body fluid. It is in the coatings that protect cell membranes.**

When the inner lining of arteries is threatened or damaged by irritants, oxidizers and chemicals (free radicals), cholesterol accumulates and creates a protective coating.

The need for cholesterol is second only to proteins and calcium. It is an oil type substance produced mainly by the liver, as well as in minute quantities by almost every cell in the body. If we do not include enough cholesterol in our daily diet to provide the brain, nerves, blood and cells with their need, the liver compensates and creates from other body biochemicals, the amounts of cholesterol required to furnish all body needs.

The brain cannot function without generous amounts of cholesterol. Up to 17 percent of the biochemicals that make up brain matter is cholesterol. Cholesterol is one of the components that forms the outer coatings of nerves called the "myelin sheaths". Like a suit of armor, these sheaths protect nerves from harm. They stop electric nerve currents from jumping from one nerve to another – from short-circuiting with other nerves. It plays a role in the metabolism of a multitude of body biochemicals and functions. It is an essential building block of blood. Cholesterol is a part of blood, mother's milk, kidneys and adrenal glands.

It is one of the basic building materials in the formation of male, female and adrenal hormones. In conjunction with the rays of the sun, cholesterol is a key factor in the formation of Vitamin D by the under-layers of the skin.

Cholesterol is essential for the fabrication of bile – a major and indispensable body detoxifier. Eighty percent of cholesterol is used in and by the liver to do this.

Cholesterol is an essential compound of biological membranes and a precursor of glucocorticoids, mineralcorticoids, sexual hormones, Vitamin D and bile acids. Cholesterol is found in animal fats, blood, nerve tissue, and bile. It is essential to your health. Your liver or intestines produces from 66 to 85 percent of the cholesterol it needs. The disadvantage about cholesterol is that it can become responsible for blockages that cause arteriosclerosis and heart attacks, in addition to a host of illnesses. But that is only part of the story. You need cholesterol and all the good things it can do for you. Here is a list of the critical benefits of cholesterol:

1. Aids in carbohydrate metabolism.
2. Helps the skin convert the sun's ultraviolet rays into the essential Vitamin D.
3. Main supplier of adrenal steroid hormones, for example cortisone.
4. Critical part of every membrane and required for the making of sex hormones.
5. Cholesterol is transported through the blood stream by hitching a ride and bonding with proteins. Three main varieties of protein are used by cholesterol for its transportation in the blood system. They are:

   1) Low-density lipoproteins (LDL)
   2) Very-low density lipoproteins (VLDL)
   3) High-density lipoproteins (HDL)

Currently it is the ratio between LDL and HDL that is used to determine whether or not you have a healthy balance.

- The overall percentages of these proteins in the system is as follows LDL (65%) VLDL (15%) and HDL (20%).
- Studies indicate that HDL, which is made up mainly of the very important fat lecithin, is the blood systems' internal scrubber that breaks up and prevents the plaque byproducts of LDL from causing arterial blockages.

The table below shows risk categories and target lipid levels pertaining to levels of LDL cholesterol levels and total cholesterol: HDL cholesterol.

Patients at high risk include those with established coronary artery disease CAD, cerebrovascular disease or peripheral arterial disease; patients with chronic kidney disease; adult diabetes patients; and asymptomatic patients in whom the 10-year risk of death from CAD or non-fatal myocardial infarction is 20 percent or higher. Patients at moderate (intermediate) risk include those with a 10-year risk greater than 10 percent but less than 20 percent.

**Target level**

| Risk category | LDL-C level mmol/L | TC:HDL-C ratio |
|---|---|---|
| High* (10-year risk of coronary artery disease 20%, or history of diabetes mellitus** or any atherosclerotic disease) | < 2.5 and | < 4.0 |
| Moderate (10-year risk 11%–19%) | < 3.5 and | < 5.0 |
| Low*** (10-year risk 10%) | < 4.5 and | < 6.0 |

Source: CMAJ • 28 OCT. 2003; 169 (9)

There are also risk factors to consider when dealing with cardiovascular problems as indicated by the table below:

- **Risk factors for heart disease and stroke**

| Age | Gender |
|---|---|
| Family history | Tobacco smoking |
| Physical inactivity | High blood pressure |
| Dyslipidemia | Overweight |
| Diabetes | Excessive alcohol use |
| Hyperhomocysteinemia | Oxidant diet/Antioxidant use |
| Mental Stress | Exertion in the cold/Snow shoveling |
| Infections and inflammatory agents | Atrial fibrillation |
| Ethnicity | |

Source: The Changing Face of Heart Disease and Stroke in Canada

## There is no cholesterol disease or health problem.

To consider cholesterol as an undesirable substance or a hazard to health is completely misleading; without good, normal, healthy cholesterol, we could not live for 30 seconds. Abnormal cholesterol is a different story. It is a serious body hazard and can cause a number of ailments.

Misinformation about cholesterol, oils and fats confuses people and influences the masses to not include quality oils that they seriously need in their diets. The food cartels and media persuade the public to buy and use cheap, refined, chemically processed harmful oils, margarines, salad dressings, sandwich spreads, fried foods and chips. Possibly, the worst of oils is mineral oil. It can react with and destroy the body's normal oils. Ultimately, it strongly contributes and predisposes cancer.

The food companies are now selling foods with synthetic oil (olestra), which depletes our bodies of its normal oils and adds to a real cholesterol problem and has cancer causing properties. Most of these commercial, refined and processed "non-cholesterol" foods are far more harmful than quality cholesterol foods. They upset and block the body's ability to effectively utilize cholesterol.

Contrary to the promotional scares of the drug companies, medics and food industries research on cholesterol has proven...

"There is no relationship between the amount of cholesterol and unsaturated oils you eat and the incidence of heart disease. Eskimos eat huge amounts of fats and oils. Eighty percent of heart patients have normal cholesterol levels." *Framingham Report* 1970 – Doctors W. Kannel and T. Gordon.

***There never has been scientific proof that lowering blood (normal) cholesterol levels prevents heart disease.***

"Unsaturated oils and healthy cholesterol in the diet are not the cause of coronary heart disease. That myth is the greatest scientific deception of the century, perhaps of any century." George V. Mann, M.D., Prof. of Medicine and Biochemistry, Vanderbilt University, 1991.

~~~~

"High blood cholesterol levels are not acceptable or reliable predictors of heart and other disease risk. Blood cholesterol levels vary greatly – even throughout the day. Simply varying the position of the body when blood is taken can alter test findings." *American Family Physician, September 1986.*

~~~~

"The complications of high blood cholesterol are related, but little, to the amount ingested in the body in the form of good quality food. Doubling or tripling food intake only mildly increases the blood cholesterol levels." Dr. Keys – Science 112:79.

Cholesterol fanatics warn us to stay away from eggs, because they are rich in cholesterol. Only eggs from unhealthy chicken, chickens raised on unhealthy feed are high in abnormal cholesterol.

Healthy, fertilized eggs from range fed chickens contain high levels of lecithin and other elements, which rapidly and effectively metabolize cholesterol. They lower the levels of cholesterol in the blood wherever it is high.

~~~~

"All studies we have done showed no effect (on blood cholesterol) of high egg consumption in a normal diet." - Margaret Flynn, Clinical Dietitian, University of Missouri in Columbia

~~~~

There is no relationship between blood cholesterol levels and hardening of arteries. A chemical called "homocysteine", rather than cholesterol, is the agent that hardens arteries and creates disease.

~~~~

"Homocysteine is a toxic substance regularly produced from methionine. It remains toxic, if not converted to cystethionine by the action of Vitamin B6. Vitamin B6 is plentiful in fruits and vegetables; it is low in meats and dairy products." Dr. K McCully, Howard Medical School.

At best, blood cholesterol levels are but rough indicators of various diseases.

**Abnormal cholesterol, toxic fats and toxic oils are the problem**. They are serious threats to our health. Cholesterol creates only health benefits and offers no problem.

## A real (abnormal) cholesterol problem originates from three sources:

- Excess intakes of fats, toxic oils and denatured cholesterol.
- The commercial, chemical distorting and denaturing of cholesterol and dietary oils.
- The body's inability to detoxify and eliminate abnormal cholesterol.

### Fats versus Oils

Fats are not oils. Fats are different from oils as black is from white. Because chemistry books call both fats and oils "unsaturated fatty acids" oils are often referred to as fats. At room temperatures, oils are liquid and fats are solid. There is no resemblance between the ways each act and react. To confuse oils with fats is a serious mistake.

All fatty tissues are made up of fat cells which have become storage deposits and garbage pails for body wastes, poisons, toxins, wastes and excesses that the body cannot use.

Fat is unhealthy toxic tissue. It is always a hazard to health. Fats contain generous amounts of abnormal toxic cholesterol. They can contribute more than any foods to high blood cholesterol levels.

However, fats do have some value. By storing body wastes and keeping useless and hazardous substances from overloading the blood, fat tissues prevent these from overloading and congesting our organs and from interfering with the normal healthy chemical reactions of body metabolism. Fat tissue obviously adds to body beauty by creating its soft lines and contours. However, fats are best not used as foods. Fats in foods create fats in our bodies.

## Fat and Abnormal Cholesterol Sources:

- All prepared meats, like salami, bologna, canned meats, hot dogs and sausages.
- High-fat cheeses, cream and processed cheeses.
- Red meats: even meat that appears lean contains up to 18 percent fat. Before cooking and eating, trim off visible fat.
- Shellfish: clams, crab, lobster, oysters, scallops, and shrimp. These are all high in cholesterol and lack the oils and enzymes for cholesterol metabolism.
- Barbecue to meats: the high heat turns the melted fat drippings that drop into the hot coals, into rancid toxic, cancer causing fats. These rise in the smoke fumes and saturate the meats.
- Tuna and salmon in cans: the cans are put to a very high heat of a prolonged period of time. This heat destroys all nutrient values. Any food value still remaining is not enough to nourish the jaw muscles as they chew these foods.
- Fresh tuna and salmon are still valuable foods if boiled and eaten fresh. Broiling melts the fats, which can then be poured off.
- The only quality sardines are those packed in their own oils. Sardines packed in oils other than their own, are not recommended.
- Commercial buns, rolls, biscuits, donuts, sweet rolls, cheese breads, muffins, cakes, mixes, batters and foods containing commercial egg yolks.
- Gravies and sauces are rich in cholesterol and fat.
- The commercial grocery store "assembly-line" produced eggs are "sick" eggs. Sick eggs are loaded with abnormal cholesterol. They lack normal lecithin and enzymes required by the body to use and metabolize this cholesterol. Even a small number of sick eggs will add to blood cholesterol levels.
- Pasteurized milk and yogurt, and products made from pasteurized milk. The fat content of skim milk may be

tolerable, but regular and homogenized, pasteurized milk have too much fat and enzyme to help your body handle it.

- Hydrogen oils:
  - o roasted nuts
  - o Stale flowers, wheat flowers, ground up flax seed, and their oils will turn rancid within 24 to 48 hours
  - o Long-time stored, crushed cereal grains and seeds
  - o High sweets and sugar sources in the diet
  - o All carbonated beverages
  - o Tea, coffee and chocolate beverages
  - o Alcohol affects cholesterol levels. Excesses alcohol affect them excessively
  - o Cigarette Smoking

## Commercial Denaturing of Oils

Abnormal cholesterols are oxidized cholesterols. Most oil rich foods, nuts, seeds and grains, have hard outer coatings or shells. To break the outer coatings or shells and crush what is inside requires great pressure. Pressure creates heat. Both the high temperatures of the press, and the exposure of the crushed materials to air, allows the air to make contact with and react with the oils. These turn the oils rancid.

Many oils are extracted from their original foods by means of solvents. Once extracted, many of the oils are refined. Refining robs them of essential nutrients and minerals.

Bottling oils in other than dark containers exposes the oils to sunlight. Sunlight also turns oils rancid. Of all of the olive oils on the market, only the "extra fine" virgin oil is properly extracted from organically grown olives. Words like "pure" and "light" are used to give the impression of quality and deceive us into believing they have not been chemically treated.

## Abnormal cholesterol is treated by faulty metabolism

Body metabolism is comparable to the burning of wood in a fire or of fuel in a motor. Faulty metabolism is when the wood does not burn properly or the gas in a car motor does not completely ignite. Inadequately combusted or burned fuels create soot or carbon.

## Faulty cholesterol metabolism results from...

- Deficiencies: (mainly) of magnesium, potassium, manganese, vanadium, chromium, zinc, selenium, Vitamin C, E, B3, B6 and folic acid.
- Inadequate dietary intake of quality oils.
- Inadequate and incomplete digestion.
- An absence of enzymes to properly and completely utilize (metabolize) oils and cholesterol. Most important of these are the pancreatic enzymes which complete oil rich food digestion and make those oils available for absorption and use by the body.
- Faulty and inadequate functioning of liver, endocrine glands, and organs that metabolize and utilize cholesterol
- Acetic acid transformed in the body into cholesterol. There are 25 steps by which this takes place. The enzyme "HMG VoA-reductase" is the catalyst that converts HMG CoA-reductase into a mevalonic acid – the form in which the acetic acid is converted into cholesterol. CoA-reductase determines how much cholesterol is produced. It is the rate limiting factor. These factors can alter cholesterol levels by as much as 100 percent.

Inadequately utilized and metabolized, toxic cholesterol, as well as chemically distorted, abnormal, cholesterol molecules, toxic fats and oils collect in blood vessels. They deposit on the inner lining of arteries and in the webs of capillaries that infiltrate through the blood vessel walls and muscles. These deposits harden and block arteries. Depending on which blood vessels are affected, their obstruction will bring on heart conditions, high blood pressure, strokes, obesity, senility and decrease of mental alertness.

Toxic abnormal cholesterol stagnates in the gallbladder. It fosters infinite infections of the gallbladder ducts, gallstones and duct obstruction.

## Miscellaneous factors that raise cholesterol levels and interfere with its metabolism...

- Stress, tensions
- Exhaustion, fatigue and burnouts
- Fears, fright, anxieties and even loud noises
- Pain
- Pregnancy
- Tranquilizers
- Cortisone-type drugs
- Excesses of Vitamin A and D tablets
- Diuretic drugs
- Drugs for medication of epilepsy
- Birth control pills and male hormones
- Epinephrine (asthma, shock) drugs
- The mere sticking a needle into your arm
- Cigarettes increase blood cholesterol levels. They damage the inner linings of blood vessels.

## Aids to Cholesterol Metabolism and Avoidance of its Excesses

- **Eat only small meals**. Serum cholesterol declines when eating eight small, snack size meals daily instead of large ones.
- Lecithin fragments and disintegrates cholesterol, fats and oils into microscopic particles in the bloodstream . They can then pass readily through the arterial walls and be readily utilized by the tissues.

  Foods rich in lecithin are the yellow of eggs, nuts, seeds and whole-grain products, liver and other organ meats.

  Lecithin in supplement form must not be processed, treated with chemicals, or heated. Its enzyme content must be intact. An ideal supplement form is a paste consistency type lecithin in a perle form. When lecithin intake is inadequate, the excesses of cholesterol foods and of hydrogenated oils may increase the cholesterol levels in the blood. The late Dr. Lawrence Kinsell, found that lecithin "lowers blood cholesterol profoundly."

- **Natural, quality, unrefined oils** – two to three tablespoons taken daily, aid normal cholesterol utilization
- **Beet juice and Black radish** (standard process), supplements, olive leaves, artichokes, watercress are rich sources of **liver flushing enzymes**. They help rid blood cholesterol excesses.
- **Bile**(in capsules) is fat solubilizing and emulsifying.
- **Livers cell extracts and tonics.** The liver is the organ which makes, uses and metabolizes cholesterol. In a cholesterol problem, it is the first organ to be checked, supported and cared for.
- **Periodic liver flushes** – two ounces of oil in a glass of citrus juice.
- **Apples:** they are rich in pectin. Pectin helps lower blood cholesterol levels.
- **Herbs:** burdock and milk thistle
- **Fiber roughage** increases cholesterol metabolism
- **Exercise:** a great tension release or an activator of blood flow to and from all tissues
- **Rest, relaxation** release from tensions, and stresses

**Effects and side effects of drug medications to lower cholesterol:**

- No drugs effectively lower cholesterol
- Mechanisms of actions are undefined
- They also alter the other normal oils in the body
- Cataracts. R. Cenedella, PhD, Liver Disease in the *Journal of American Medical Association*, March 27, 1987
- Cancer (stomach/intestines)Dr. Pinckney Lancet
- Constipation
- Calcification or colics of the gallbladder
- Hemorrhoids
- Hemorrhages from stomach ulcers

- Pancreatitis (inflammation of the pancreas)
- Anemia
- Shortness of breath – asthma
- Dizziness – fainting
- Headaches
- Anxiety
- Intestinal gas, bloating, flatulence
- Nausea, diarrhea
- Accidents, death from hardening of brain arteries

If your doctor prescribes an anti-cholesterol drug for you, ask him why he does not also prescribe a diet and a lifestyle for lowing cholesterol.

Naturopathic medicine can complement other medical disciplines to attain optimum health with dietary interventions. Dietary management of LDL-C is the major goal of coronary heart disease (CHD) risk management. The principal strategy for lowering LDL-C is to replace cholesterol-raising fatty acids (i.e. saturated and *trans*fatty acids) with carbohydrates and/or unsaturated fatty acids. Therefore, the AMERICAN HEART ASSOCIATION (2006), recommends switching to a diet low in saturated fat (7 % of total calories) and dietary cholesterol (200 mg/d) as the first stage therapeutic cholesterol-lowering measure in primary prevention of CHD.

Changing the diet in this way may reduce LDL-C by around 11-16 percent - possibly as much as 20 percent. Several clinical studies have proven such an effect, as the following references demonstrate:

- LDL-C lowering can be enhanced by increasing dietary intake of soluble fiber (recommendation 10-25 g/day). An increase in fiber from 5 to 10 g/d is expected to reduce LDL-C by 3 to 5 percent.
- The mechanisms by which fiber helps to decrease serum cholesterol are not yet fully understood.
- It is suggested that soluble fiber binds bile acids or cholesterol during intraluminal formation of micelles. The

resulting reduction of cholesterol in hepatic cells leads to an up-regulation of LDL receptors and thus to increased clearance of LDL-cholesterol. Moreover, products of fiber fermentation may inhibit fatty acid synthesis (BROWN ET AL. 1999).

- In addition, soy can lower LDL-C by about 5 percent (FLETCHER ET AL. 2005). There appear to be several lipid-lowering mechanisms involved. Soy consumption is believed to increase the secretion of cholecystokinin and stimulate bile acid synthesis.

- As estrogens are known to lower LDL-C, it is also possible that the LDL-C decrease is a result of the estrogenic effects of soy (ERDMAN ET AL. 2000).

- Finally, it is evident that plant sterols and plant stanols decrease total and LDL-cholesterol by up to 15 percent. Several health organizations such as the American Heart Association and the American Association for Clinical Nutrition recommend a supplementation of 2 g plant sterol/stanol per day as a cholesterol-lowering therapeutic option.

Nutritional interventions may have cumulative effects as a result of their different cholesterol-lowering mechanisms. JENTKINS ET AL. (2003) demonstrated that the LDL-C reduction of 28.6 percent induced by a low-fat diet (-8 %) was the result of consuming foods high in viscous fiber, soy protein, almonds and plant sterols. Such a diet therefore appears to produce a similar LDL-C lowering effect to that of an initial dose of a first-generation statin (-30.9 percent).

Analyzing the long term (1-year) effect of a low fat diet rich in fiber, almonds, soy and plant sterols, over 30 percent of motivated patients were able to lower their LDL-C by more than 20 percent. (JENTKINS ET AL. 2006)

**Nutritional factors lowering LDL-C (GRUNDY 2006) can be seen below:**

| Appropriate Reduction (CVD) | LDL-C Reduction |
|---|---|
| Saturated fat – 7% | 8-10% |
| Dietary Cholesterol 200 mg/dl – 3% | 3-5% |
| Dietary Fiber – 3% | 3-5% |
| Plant Sterols/Stanols – 6% | 5-15% |
| Soy Protein | 5% |
| CUMULATIVE | 20-30% |

## Cholesterol balance is essential

Too much as well as too little cholesterol can create an imbalance. Excess cholesterol is less of a problem than deficiencies of cholesterol.

*Low blood cholesterol* levels increase incidences of cancer, gallbladder problems, aggressiveness, violent behaviors, personality disturbances, homicide, suicide, irresponsibility, and poor self-control and body aging.

Your body senses when it is deficient in cholesterol. It will maintain constant blood levels of cholesterol regardless of the amount of cholesterol taken into our bodies in our diet.

The body protects itself readily from its low levels in a number of ways. Your liver, muscles, skin and all cells produce cholesterol.

These may overcompensate and even produce more than normal amounts. Together, they can and will synthesize, daily nearly 1600 to 1700 mg of cholesterol.

## Food preparing to avoid toxic cholesterol

- Cook foods by baking, broiling or steaming. Never put food onto the top of the stove if it can be conveniently cooked inside an oven.
- Always undercook foods. Do not cook to the point that the flavor, color, consistency is radically changed.

## Cholesterol Myths

Mistaken notions about cholesterol are admirably discussed by Dr. W. Gifford- Jones, M.D. in his book, *The Doctor Game*. The following summarizes his comments.

"It has been said, it's not what you don't know that gets you into trouble, it is what you know for sure that ain't so. Many things about cholesterol "ain't so." The drug and food companies, aided and abetted by the medical profession, have created "cholesterol phobia"

"The only way to eliminate this insidious phobia is to disencumber one's self of 12 myths."

**Myth # 1:** The only way the body obtains cholesterol is by consuming it. Not so. About 80 percent of cholesterol in the human body is produced by the liver. Following dietary measures does little to decrease blood cholesterol. Altering our internal metabolism is as difficult as trying to change the spots on a leopard.

**Myth # 2:** The more cholesterol we eat, the greater the amount will be in the blood. Not so. Studies show that the more cholesterol consumed, the less the liver produces, the absorption of cholesterol decreases and the excretion of cholesterol increases. If the diet is low in cholesterol, the liver gets the message to produce increased amounts.

**Myth # 3:** A single blood test is an accurate way to determine the level of blood cholesterol. It is a fallacy to place so much faith in a laboratory results. Studies show that laboratories have reported results that are as much as 15 percent either too high or too low.

Erroneous results can cause either needless worry or a false sense of security. Several tests are normally required to obtain a reliable figure.

**Myth # 4:** Precise blood test results can predict whether or not a coronary attack will occur. Not so. Coronary attacks are caused much more by stress, tension, lifestyle excesses, blood circulation problems, then by cholesterol. Abnormal cholesterol levels only add to our predisposition to a heart attack that already exists.

**Myth #5:** Dietary cholesterol is the primary risk factor for coronary disease. It is unrealistic to believe that only one factor is responsible for heart troubles (or for any disease). Genetics, diabetes, hypertension, smoking, lack of exercise, inadequate fibrous intake, high fat diet, obesity and advancing age are important risk factors. The amounts of toxic oils and the toxic substances in oils do more to cause heart disease than do the blood cholesterol levels.

**Myth #6:** Low blood cholesterol levels guarantee that hardening of the arteries will not occur. Not so. Dr. Michael Debakey, a famous Texas heart surgeon, reports that 30 percent of patients, who have a coronary bypass, have normal blood cholesterol.

**Myth #7:** Similar blood cholesterol levels trigger a similar number of heart attacks. Not so. Cholesterol levels of males living in Edinburgh and Stockholm are nearly identical, but the coronary deaths for the Scottish are three times higher than the Swedish.

**Myth #8**: Dairy products should be avoided. They increase blood cholesterol and trigger atherosclerosis. Nonsense. (Healthy) eggs are a good source of protein, iron, phosphorus and Vitamin A and are low in saturated oils (fats). Blaming hens and cows for coronary disease is like accusing the iceberg for sinking the Titanic. Heart attacks result from faulty and foolish lifestyles and diets.

**Myth #9:** Chemical and drug companies are user-friendly and have your wellbeing at heart. You are being naïve and live in

Never, Never Land if you believe this one. Corporations deceive consumers in many ways. Some companies advertise their products as "cholesterol free" when in fact at no time did they ever contain any. They load their products with sugar (some breakfast cereals contain as much as 50 percent sugar) salt, additives and preservatives, which, like many foods that don't contain cholesterol, create biochemical conditions which make the cholesterol levels increase.

Whatever nutrients the foods from which the cereals are prepared, they have been so destroyed by their methods of preparation that there is no food value in their contents. It is healthier to eat the boxes.

**Myth #10:** Drugs are the best way to decrease elevated blood cholesterol levels. Not so. Nothing is that simple. There is no such thing as a non-toxic, harmless drug. Molière, the French playwright, remarked in 1673 that nearly all men die of their medicines, not of their diseases. It still happens today. It's impossible to take cholesterol lowering medication for years without side effects. It makes more sense to correct and eliminate the causes and the faulty lifestyle.

**Myth #11:** The best way to attack the cholesterol problem is to run cholesterol tests on everyone. Protect us, Lord, from this folly. It will waste millions of dollars, scare people half to death and increase the epidemic of cholesterol phobia.

**Myth #12:** All cholesterol rich foods are harmful and overload our bodies with cholesterol.

Unprocessed, unrefined, quality cholesterol rich foods contain enzymes and biochemical agents our bodies need to utilize and take advantage of the cholesterol those foods contain.

## Marvels, benefits and need for quality oil

Oils are essential nutrients, as essential as any nutrient. After protein, oils are next of importance. Oils, like cholesterol, are vital components of all cell membranes.

Misconceptions and theories about calories of fats and oils have induced most to restrict oils. Your body cannot create oils. It must get them from foods. It must get them regularly, daily, and in generous quantities. We generally and daily need about two tablespoons of oil or oil rich foods. Bodies seemingly have an unlimited ability to burn and use oils. It is difficult to get too much oil in one's diet.

More people lack quality oils in their diets and bodies than vitamins, minerals or proteins. A diet that deprives our bodies of oils is a criminal offense against our bodies.

Oils are better digested and more easily assimilated when in combination with the proteins of the foods, like seeds, nuts and grains, in which they originally existed. According to tests done on animals, high protein diets, in the absence of oils, cause severe deficiency and obesity.

Our tissues cannot use oils that have been denatured, chemically treated, that are rancid or have been changed in any way. Including generous amounts of quality oils help to burn up or get rid of the abnormal ones.

When our bodies do not succeed in handling or eliminating toxic oils, they store them in fatty tissues. Excesses create obesity. However, one of the worst mistakes an obese person can make is to cut out quality oils, believing and expecting that this will prevent weight gain, or help weight loss. The contrary is true.

### *Oils are our greatest cell protectors and safeguards against disease. Oils act as cell "Suits of Armor".*

One of the greatest injustices of the presentations of counsels and guidelines to health and living is the failure to inform everybody of the wonders and importance of oils.

## Without oils:

- Bodies would not be able to metabolize or properly use calcium.
- Our bodies would be deprived of and seriously deficient in the oil soluble vitamins.
- The structure and strength of our bones would deteriorate. This is commonly seen in menopause when the female hormone level drops and the bones become osteoporosis.
- Nerves would function chaotically out of control.
- We would live on levels of fatigue and lethargy.
- Thyroid, adrenal (stress glands), and male/female glands would produce only low quality hormones. Oils are the raw materials from which our endocrine glands manufacture hormones. Sterols is a shortened chemical way of writing "steroids-oils".
- Livers could not perform their thousands of functions.

## *There are over 60 indispensable health-creating and restoring roles of quality oils.*

- Oils are major protectors against body wastes, toxins, poisons, pollutants, irritants, radiation, damages and diseases by forming a coating around cells. Protecting cell membranes is protecting cell health.
- The flow of nutrients into cells and the pouring out of its poisons is proportional to the amounts of oils in the membranes.

## Quality Oils...

- Defend against the hazards and effects of rancid hydrogenated, chemically denatured oils.
- Burn up and rid our bodies of toxic and counterfeit oils and fats.
- Form part of the blood carrier system that transports oxygen to cells.

- Are essential, indispensable agents that make possible cell utilization of oxygen.
- Combine with proteins to make up hemoglobin and form the body's oxygen transport system.
- Part of the metabolism that converts proteins into sources of energy.
- Create reserves of energy and stamina and endurance.
- Offset fatigue caused by low blood sugar.
- Fuel cells with the ions and energies they need in order to burn up sugars.
- Essential components and activators of the oil soluble vitamin complexes of the A, D, E and F groups.
- Make soluble, available and utilizable to our cells the same essential oil soluble A, D, E, and F vitamins.
- Essential components of normal, healthy cholesterol. Oils promote and normalize its production. They prevent the production and hazards of abnormal cholesterol.
- Prevent the buildup of triglycerides in blood and counteract their threat to heart, arteries and health.
- Protect blood vessels and arteries from hardening.
- Help give beauty shapes to bodies, filling and rounding bones and angular shapes – especially in women.
- Beautify and preserve complexion and keep it soft, supple, healthy – especially in women.
- Lubricate dry skin and keep it moist.

## Quality Oils...

- Relieve and cure "oily" scalp and dandruff.
- Play a major role in curing eczema, psoriasis and other skin diseases and conditions.
- Provide fuel for body heat, comfort and protection from the cold.
- Sustain and promote liver functions. They provide the energies, life forces, nutrients and chemical agents by

which the liver fulfills its multitudes of functions. The liver cannot function without oils.

- Stimulate the liver and gallbladder to empty their toxins and detoxified wastes into the intestines.
- Slow down liver overloading by fats and body wastes.
- Help restore fertility. Fertility is oil dependent.
- Are hormone-building materials for pituitary, adrenal, thyroid and sex gland hormones.
- Activate the pituitary gland which, in turn, acts on the thyroid and adrenal glands, and incite them to produce more of their hormones.
- Activate hormones to release fats from fatty tissues.
- Act as fat carriers. They transport fat to the liver for processing and eliminating from the body.
- Coat the walls of the intestines. This coating blocks passage of toxic and abnormal substances into bodies.
- Lubricate and facilitate the passage of fecal matter. They act as a laxative.
- Aids elimination by softening and moisturizing stools.

## Quality Oils...

- Burn up tissue fats faster than exercises, sweating or hot baths. The more fat, and the longer that fat has been with you, the better and quicker you will dissolve it by increasing your intake of oils.
- Help control appetite and stop food cravings.
- Activate body to use and to derive benefits from calcium, (not possible without the actions of oils).
- Help steady, control and calm nerves.
- Reduce sensitivities and irritabilities
- Oils provide twice the calories of sugars and carbohydrates. Using oils in the diet bypasses the body's needs from these sources of sugar.
- Help control and limit the production of excess insulin. Oils do not need nor create a need for insulin. If you have deprived yourself of oils for years, your body, in revenge,

demands twice as much sweets, sugars and carbohydrates to make up for the deficiency of this body food and fuel.

- Lubricate our joints and promote their smooth function and mobility.
- Prevent joint pains and pain-causing calcium deposits.
- Oils preclude the need for vaccinations.
- Help build immunity and protect against colds, flues and infections.
- Facilitate withdrawal from alcohol and dependence.
- A remedy for relieving stomach ulcers.
- Stop the bleeding of hemophilia. Sesame oil is a unique source of Vitamin T, the vitamin which promotes the proliferation of blood platelets that control bleeding that is otherwise uncontrollable.

## Special Oils with Special Values

- Sesame oil is rich in lecithin, which helps nerves and nerve cells. It contains sesamol, a natural anti-rancidity protector.
- The oils from primrose, borage and black currant and amaranth seeds are rich in, Gamma Linolenic acid, a special oil that does not need the action of digestive enzymes to help assimilate it into our bodies.

## Gamma Linolenic Acid (GLA) helps:

- Allergies, arthritis, arterial sclerosis
- Diabetes, obesity, premenstrual syndrome
- Alcoholism, colitis, liver degeneration
- Depressions, cancer, multiple sclerosis
- Psoriasis, eczema, skin lesions and disorders and other conditions listed in the previous pages
- Pumpkin Seed Oil is one of the most nutritious of all oils. It helps heal stomach, intestines and prostate problems and helps improve blood circulation and protects against tooth decay.

- Flax seed oil. It is possibly the richest source of the most valuable oil fractions called Omega-3.

## Flax Seed Meal

Flax seeds are rich in a component called "lignan". Lignans protect against fungi, viruses and cancer, particularly cancers of the breast, colon, prostate, uterus and ovaries.

One daily tablespoon flax seed, finally ground, provides this protection.

The coatings (outer shells) of these oil rich seeds provide possibly the finest of fibers.

The whole ground flax seed powder is also rich in vitamins, calcium, magnesium, zinc, iron, manganese, phosphate, niacin, pantothenic acid, riboflavin, thiamine and beta-carotene.

## Quality, Desirable Oils and Oil Sources

Oils are products of plants in contrast to fats which are from animal tissues.

Variety in oils is essential – as is variety of other foods. Each type of oil provides different types of oil components.

Oil mixtures that are valuable: Flax seed oil with sunflower oil; Sesame with olive oil. Unsalted butter mixed with other quality oils. Butter should be used sparingly.

Soy and olive oils contain the least quality or variety of oil.

**Nuts:** Almonds, hazel, pecans, walnuts, peanuts. Nuts should be fresh, shelled, unroasted and unsalted.

**Seeds:** Sesame, sunflower, safflower, flax, corn oil, soybean, wheat germ, and their oils.

**Vegetables:** Avocados

**Beans:** Chickpeas, garbanzo beans, soybeans, tofu, cornmeal and lentils

**Fish:** Salmon, cod and halibut

**Meats:** Liver, sweetbreads, internal organs

## Oils and Oil Enzymes

The oil type enzymes act like spark plugs and car cylinders, or flames in a fireplace. Oils and their enzymes transform cholesterol into cell components and into hormones. Special cholesterol utilizing enzymes are normally found in fresh, alive, quality oil and lecithin containing foods.

## All oils need special care

All oils go rancid. Rancidity is oxidized oils. Contact with the oxygen of the air oxidizes them. When they go stale, they turn rancid. Rancidity renders oils unfit for human consumption. Some, like wheat germ, flax seed oils, go rancid rapidly, within days.

Heating oils at high temperatures destroy the oil enzymes. The higher the temperature, the more rapidly and totally oils turn rancid.

## Rancid – Toxic Oils

Of all foods, rancid oils are the most toxic. Fats, chemically processed fats, lard, Crisco and shortenings are all equal in toxicity to rancid oils. Even the body wastes and excesses that get stored in fats are not nearly as toxic as rancid oils. The only substances more toxic and harmful are chemicals and drugs.

- Rancid oils are a known cause of cancer.
- Stale rancid oils act in the body in much the same ways as do fats. They interfere with and block the health promoting and protecting functions of normal oils. They usurp the place of normal oils in the body.
- Rancid oils cannot absorb into and become part of the substance of the cell membranes. Cells lose their protective coating against all attackers and hazards. Rancid oils then harm and poison those cells.

- Rancid oils block normal body oils from becoming transformed into hormones.
- Rancid oils block the functions and healing properties of oil soluble vitamins.
- Rancid oils, hydrogenated oils, margarines, fried foods, peanut butters and spreads, prevent the normal utilization and metabolism of cholesterol.
- An excessive amount of oil predominantly from any one of kind fatty acid, create an imbalance.

## Factors that destroy oils (turn them rancid)

- Milling of grains and seeds - extracting the germ.
- Discarding the germs of seeds that contain the oils.
- Extracting the oils and exposing them to chemicals, air, sunlight and radiation.
- Food production practices. Growing animals, chickens and fish in caged conditions and feeding them with the cheapest and poor quality foods (according to the choice of the growers) has decreased the contents of those foods to as much as 1/5 normal levels.
- Hydrogenation. Replacing oxygen by hydrogen blocks the rancidification of oils. This process also eliminates the foul taste and odor of oxygenated oils. This fools the public into believing that the oils they are buying and using are still fresh and good quality.
- This is "hydrogenation". Hydrogenation is used to thicken and stabilize oils, like in the making of margarine, creamy peanut butters, different dressings and spread. Hydrogen combines with oils in the same way as oxygen. The oils don't go rancid. However, the hydrogen denatures and destroys the oils in ways worse than rancidity.
- Hydrogenated oils, like fats, are rich in abnormal, denatured cholesterol. They markedly aggravate cholesterol problems. They hinder the production of normal hormones and deprive the cells of their protective

coatings. Hydrogenation is the worst atrocity perpetrated on foods.

- Combining oils with drugs, chemicals and toxic foods. Aspirin blocks the availability of body ability to use oils. Sugar, coffee, junk foods, refined carbohydrates and the chemical additives in foods do the same.
- Viral infections
- Chemical denaturing: even science doesn't completely know all the chemical reactions which take place in our bodies nor which body pollutants or toxins react with oils and cholesterol. But we know that it is not possible for two incompatible chemicals to encounter each other without a mutually destroying reaction taking place.

Any and all abnormal chemicals have an affinity for enzymes. When you destroy the enzymes that are part of the oil complexes, you destroy the ability of those oils, as well as cholesterols, to function in their normal health giving ways.

Marketing oils with chemical preservatives: there is no such substance or chemical that can be rightfully called a preservative. They act on foods in the same way that "preservative" embalming fluids undertakers inject into your veins, will act on you when you are a corpse. Quality oils are almost nonexistent at ordinary grocery stores.

- Washing and bathing with soaps. Every soap dissolves and takes out oils from your skin. Use only oil-based soaps (like the old-fashioned Palmolive), or those available at health stores.

## Precautions and Don'ts

- It is advisable to avoid the standard, commercial and grocery store brands of salad oils, mayonnaise. (Kraft, Heinz, etc.)
- Once oil bottles are opened, do not leave them exposed to the air or to room temperatures. Do not store them in

refrigerators. The high humidity of refrigerators also provokes rancidity.

- Store oils only in freezers. Some oils will solidify. When oil is needed, place the bottle or container under a hot water tap. Melt the quantity you intend to use. Pour it into the food you are eating. Return the oil the freezer.
- Do not fry foods or use oils in the frying unless frying is done at slow, low temperatures – just enough to heat the foods – like Chinese wok cooking, which only minimally changes the nature of the foods.

## Protecting oils against oxygen distraction

We breathe in up to 1500 pounds of air each day. Ten percent of the air, up to 150 pounds, is pure oxygen. It seems impossible to conceive that anything in our blood or our bodies can escape being oxygenated, especially our oils and oil soluble foods. The body has a protective barrier against the effects of oxygen. It uses as anti-oxidants, alpha tocopherols, which are part of the Vitamin E complex.

## Toxic Oils and Toxic Cholesterol Excesses

Some chemicals react in ways similar to oxygen. Preservatives, food additives, pollutants and drugs, act on and denature oils in ways equal to or worse than the actions of oxygen, rancidity or hydrogenation. One of the worst enemies of oils is chlorine and members of the chlorine family. The bleaching by chlorine is chemical oxidation. Chlorine bleaches foods the same as it bleaches clothes. Bleaching destroys whatever foods or substances it attacks. The amount of chlorine in drinking water is sufficient to do this.

The following sources of fat toxicities are just as toxic and contribute just as much to our health problems and are to be carefully avoided:

- All commercially fried and deep fried foods – French fries, corn and potato chips, fish and chips meals.

- All pork products: ham, bacon, pork sausages etc. most pork foods can contain up to 50 percent fat (toxins).
- Fatty and greasy foods and fats of meats: duck and goose
- Margarines: the harder the margarine, the more the oils have been hydrogenated – including soya margarines sold in health stores.
- Coconut oils and foods and candles which contain these are high in saturated oils. What we buy in grocery stores is rancid or chemically prepared.
- All oils which have been used for cooking get heated at high temperatures. Never cook twice with the same oil.
- Cottonseed oils. It is usually high in DDT.
- Cream substitutes and artificial whip creams. Ice cream, sundaes and chocolate milks.
- Crisco, shortening, lards and cooking fats.
- Salted butter. One never knows how long it has been stored. If stored too long, it is rancid.
- All processed, standard-store-style sandwich spreads, mayonnaises and salad dressings.
- Oils packaged in clear transparent bottles. Light rays can denature the oils as much as oxygen does.

## Conclusions

- Oils are a most valuable part of the body makeup – its cells, its functions, its stability and integrity.
- Oils are essential to functioning of those organs responsible for sustaining our life and protecting us from diseases.
- Oils help us avoid and protect us against 27 symptoms and 59 diseases. To not have a daily intake of oils leaves us prone to any of these conditions.
- Quality oil Deficiencies are a definite health hazard. Any publications that condemn oils or any promotion of diets that deprive our bodies of its oils are criminal offenses against our bodies.

- The final key to the role of all oils, fats and cholesterol is balance. Too much or too little of any one can lead to health problems and disease.
- Considering the great importance of oils and fats health, only a surprisingly small amount of good literature has been published.

# Glossary of Herbs

The following are popular herbs to consider managing hypoglycemia, high blood pressure and high cholesterol. As always, please discuss with your holistic practitioner.

## *Vitisvinifera* (Grape Berry, Seed)

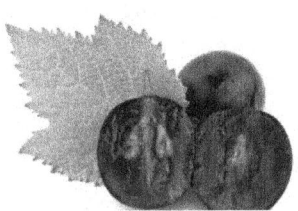 Semen VitisViniferae (grape seed) extract is a natural rich source of the bioflavonoids commonly known as procyanidins, both in quantity and variety (Santos-Buelga et al., 1995; Agarwal et al., 2002). Procyanidins are a class of polyphenolic compounds composed of flavan-3-ol subunits (oligomers and polymers (Fine, 2000). Grape seed extract (GSE) has been reported to possess a broad spectrum of pharmacological and therapeutic effects such as anti-oxidative, anti-inflammatory, antimicrobial activities, antiviral activities, cardioprotective, hepatoprotective, and neuroprotective effects (Nassiri-Asl&Hosseinzadeh, 2009).

Human case reports and results from basic research provide preliminary evidence that grape seed extract (GSE) may affect diseases, hypertension, high levels of blood cholesterol, platelet aggregation, inflammation, reduce the risk for cancer, to treat diabetic retinopathy and neuropathy and various other conditions (Sravanthi et al., 2013).

## R- Lipoic acid ($C_8H_{14}O_2S_2$)

α-Lipoic acid (LA), also known as thioctic acid, is a naturally occurring compound that is synthesized in small amounts by plants and animals, including humans (Reed, 2001). Exogenous LA from can be activated with adenosine triphosphate or guanosine triphosphate by lipoate-activating enzyme, and transferred to LA-dependent enzymes by lipoyltransferase (Fujiwara et al., 1999; Fujiwara et al., 2001). Pharmacokinetic studies in humans have found that about 30%-40% of an oral dose of LA is absorbed (Teichert et al, 2003) and the maximal plasma LA concentrations were evident between 0.5 to 1 hr following an oral dose (Breithaupt-Grögler et al., 1999).

LA scavenges a variety of reactive oxygen species (ROS) and nitrogen species (RNS), chelates transition metal ions (e.g. Iron and copper), increases cytosolic glutathione and vitamin C levels and prevents toxicities associated with their loss (Smith et al., 2004). Researchers have also found LA increases intracellular coenzyme Q10 levels (Kozlov et al., 1999). Pharmacologically, LA improves glycemic control, polyneuropathies associated with diabetes mellitus, and effectively mitigates toxicities associated with heavy metal poisoning (Smith et al., 2004).

### *Vitisvinifera* (Grape Berry)

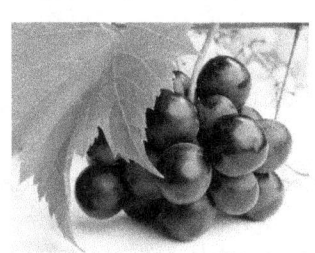

Red wine extract phenolic compounds include flavonoids and non-flavonoids (Vidavalur et al., 2006). The main type of phenolic compounds found in red wine, including hydroxybenzoic and hydroxycinnamic acids, stilbenes (eg. resveratrol), flavones, flavonols, flavanonols, flavanols, and anthocyanins (Monagas et al., 2005).

There is extensive epidemiological evidence suggesting that dietary intake of these compounds reduces cardiovascular mortality (Hertog et al., 1995). *In vivo* studies have shown that red wine intake enhanced cardio-protection and can be attributed to grape-derived polyphenols, e.g., resveratrol, in red wine (Wu & Hsieh, 2011). Red wine extract may also have a preventative effect for people at risk for type 2 diabetes (Robertson, 2014).

### *Camellia sinensis* (Green Tea, Leaf)

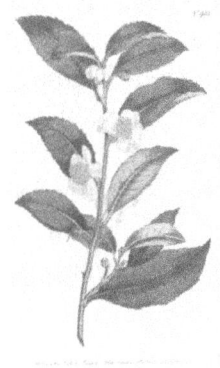

Folium Camelliae (green tea leaf) infusion is the most widely consumed beverage in the world, aside from water (Graham, 1992). The health benefits of Folium Camelliae for a wide variety of ailments, including different types of cancer, heart disease, and liver disease, have been reported. Long-term consumption of green tea could be beneficial against high-fat diet-induced obesity and type II diabetes and could reduce the risk of coronary disease (Chacko et al., 2010).

The health-promoting effects of green tea are mainly attributed to its polyphenol content known as catechins, which usually account for 30–42% of the dry weight of the solids in brewed green tea. The four major catechins include (–)-epigallocatechingallate (EGCG), (–)-epigallocatechin (EGC), (–)-epicatechingallate (ECG), and (–)-epicatechin (EC) [Mukhtar& Ahmad, 1999; Khan &Mukhtar, 2007].

### *Pinus pinaster* (Maritime Pine, Bark)

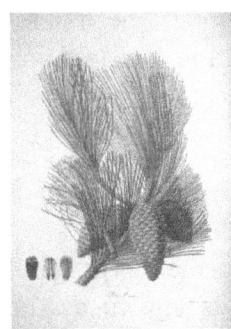

Cortex Pinus Pinaster (*Pinus pinaster* bark) extract exhibits strong free radical-scavenging activity against reactive oxygen and nitrogen species. *Pinus pinaster* bark extract (PBE) contains polyphenolic compounds such as catechin, taxifolin, procyanidins of various chain lengths formed by catechin and epicatechin units, and phenolic acids which are capable of producing diverse potentially protective effects against chronic and degenerative diseases (Rohdewald, 2005; Iravani&Zolfaghari, 2011). An increasing body of evidence indicates that PBE has favorable pharmacological properties (Rohdewald, 2002).

There are many potential uses for **PBE**, the most well-studied use is for improving vascular health as a result of improved endothelial function and venous insufficiency. Controlled clinical trials have been published that demonstrate symptomatic improvement of blood circulation, blood pressure and platelet function normalization, and venous insufficiency. Controlled clinical trials have also been published for the following indications: thrombosis, diabetes and its complications and hypertension.

### *Vacciniummyrtillus* (Bilberry, Berry)

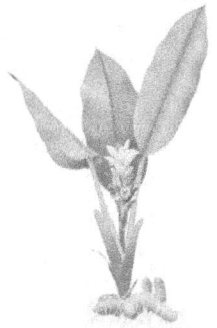

Several active constituents have been isolated from FructusVacciniMyrtilli (Bilberry berry) including anthocyanoside flavonoids (anthocyanins) and are considered the most important of the pharmacologically active compounds (Baj et al., 1983; Katsube et al., 2003; Lila, 2004). The effects of anthocyanins include antioxidant, anti-allergic, anti-inflammatory, anti-viral, anti-proliferative, anti-mutagenic, anti-microbial, anti-carcinogenic, protection from cardiovascular damage and allergy, microcirculation improvement, peripheral capillary fragility prevention, diabetes prevention, and vision improvement (Ghosh &Konishi, 2007

### *Curcuma longa* (Turmeric, Rhizome)

RhizomaCurcumaeLongae (Turmeric rhizome) contains a class of compounds known as the curcuminoids, comprised of curcumin (diferuloylmethane), demethoxycurcumin and bisdemethoxycurcumin (Jurenka, 2009). Curcumin is the principal curcuminoid and comprises 0.3–5.4 percent of raw turmeric (Akram et al., 2010); it is responsible for the yellow color of the spice as well as the majority of turmeric's therapeutic effects

(Chattopadhyay et al., 2004).

Rhizoma Curcumae Longae extracts exhibit various pharmacological activities, which include antioxidant (Sharma, 1976), anti-inflammatory (Rao et al., 1982), anti-diabetic (Mohankumar& McFarlane, 2011), anti-carcinogenic (Chen & Huang, 1998), antimutagenic (Shukla et al., 2002), antiproliferative (Mehta et al., 1997), anti-angiogenic (Gururaj et al., 2002), anticoagulant (Kim et al., 2012), antifibrotic (Punithavathi et al., 2000), antidepressant (Yu et al., 2002), antiulcer (Tuorkey& Karolin, 2009), antibacterial (Lutomski et al., 1974), antifungal (Martins et al., 2009), antiprotozoal (Rasmussen et al., 2000), antiviral (Li et al., 1993), antifertility (Mishra & Singh, 2009), hepatoprotective (Cerný et al., 2011), hypotensive (Nirmala&Puvanakrishnan, 1996), hypocholesteremic (Patil& Srinivasan, 1971), and immunomodulatory (Yue et al., 2010) properties.

Human studies have shown curcumin is rapidly metabolized, conjugated in the liver, and excreted in the feces, therefore having limited systemic bioavailability (Vareed et al., 2008).

**Inositol Hexanicotinate** (Niacin, $C_{42}H_{30}N_6O_{12}$)
Source of niacin

Hexanicotinyl cis-1,2,3,5-trans-4,6-cyclohexane (inositol hexanicotinate [IHN]) is the hexanicotinic acid ester of meso-inositol. This compound consists of six molecules of nicotinic acid (niacin) with an inositol molecule in the center. Pharmacokinetic studies indicate the IHN molecule is, at least in part, absorbed intact, and hydrolyzed in the body with release of free niacin and inositol (Harthon&Brattsand, 1979). INH is marketed as "no-flush niacin" (Benjó et al., 2006). Available data suggests that IHN does not produce a flushing reaction is consistent with the modest nicotinic acid plasma response following IHN intake (Holti, 1979; Kruse et al., 1979; Benjó et al., 2006). IHN is better tolerated and safer alternative to nicotinic acid and extended-release nicotinic acid (Head, 1996).

In 2009, the European Food Safety Authority (EFSA) Scientific Panel on Food Additives and Nutrient Sources Added to Food concluded that nicotinate from IHN is a bioavailable source of niacin (EFSA, 2009). The relatively high intestinal absorption rate (70%) and partial release of niacin from the IHN molecule after absorption should provide adequate source of niacin for the conventional nutritional functions (EFSA, 2009).

Blood flow improvements are therapeutically important in conditions resulting from peripheral vascular insufficiency, such as Raynaud's disease and intermittent claudication. IHN is prescribed in Europe as a patented drug known as Hexopal, which is therapeutically indicated for the symptomatic relief of severe intermittent claudication and Raynaud's disease (Aylward, 1979; O'Hara, 1985). The clinical research literature includes promising results from several studies on the use of IHN for improving blood flow in these conditions (Head, 1986, O'Hara et al., 1988). IHN appears to have application in the treatment of other conditions resulting from peripheral vascular insufficiency including threatened amputation from gangrene, restless legs syndrome, stasis dermatitis, hypertension, and atherosclerosis-related migraines (Welsh & Ede, 1961). IHN has also been used for the treatment of various dermatological conditions including lesions of scleroderma, acne, dermatitis herpetiformis, exfoliativeglossitis, and psoriasis (Welsh & Ede, 1961).

Therapeutically used for more than 50 years, niacin is the most effective clinically available agent for increasing high-density lipoprotein (HDL) cholesterol levels. Niacin also has beneficial effects on all known pro-atherogenic lipid parameters, including lowering LDL cholesterol, non-HDL-cholesterol and triglycerides (Carlson, 2005; Kamanna et al., 2009). Numerous epidemiological studies, both prospective and retrospective, have demonstrated that hyperlipidemia is a major risk factor for the development of atherosclerosis while elevated levels of HDL cholesterol convey cardio-protection (Wenchsler et al., 1980; Alderman et al., 1989)

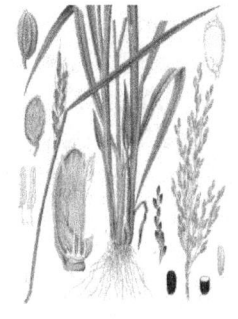

### *Monascuspurpureus- Oryza* (Red Yeast Rice, Extract) Source of monacolin K

*Monascuspurpureus*, named for its purple color, was isolated from Semen Oryzae cum MonascoFermentatum (fermented red yeast rice) in 1895 (Gordon & Becker, 2011). In 1979, Endo discovered that a strain of Monascus yeast (*Monascusruber*) naturally produced a substance that inhibits cholesterol synthesis, which he named monacolin K (Endo, 1979). European Food Safety Authority (EFSA) considers monacolin K from red yeast rice contributes to the maintenance of normal blood cholesterol concentrations (EFSA, 2011). Other active ingredients in red yeast rice include sterols (betasitosterol, campesterol, stigmasterol, sapogenin), isoflavones, and monounsaturated fatty acids (Heber et al., 1999).

Monacolin compounds are formed by *Monascus spp.* during the fermentation process. They cause a reversible competitive inhibition of the microsomal hydroxymethyl-glutaryl coenzyme A (HMG-CoA) reductase; thus, they prevent the reduction of HMG-CoA to mevalonic acid and the formation of cholesterol (Lachenmeier et al., 2012)

Red yeast rice contains monacolin K, which is chemically identical to the active ingredient in the cholesterol-lowering drug lovastatin (NCCIH, 2015) and may be a treatment option for dyslipidemic patients who cannot tolerate statin therapy (Becker et al., 2009; Halbert et al., 2010). Clinical trials have demonstrated that red yeast rice preparation reduces total cholesterol, LDL cholesterol, and total triacylglycerol concentrations in hypercholestrolemic patients (Wang et al., 1997; Heber et al., 1999). In China, consumption of red yeast rice has been studied in animals and humans and has been found to reduce cholesterol concentrations by 11–32% and triacylglycerol concentrations by 12–19% (Heber et al., 1999).

Lu et al. conducted a randomized, double-blind, placebo controlled clinical trial of 4,870 Chinese subjects over 4.5 years to evaluate the efficacy of an extract derived from red yeast rice and concluded that administration of red rice yeast extract demonstrated efficacy in decreasing cholesterol, recurrent coronary events, and mortality rates (Lu et al., 2008).

Li et al., analyzed 13 randomized, placebo-controlled trials containing 804 participants and concluded that red rice yeast exhibited significant lowering effects on serum total cholesterol and LDL cholesterol (Li et al., 2014).

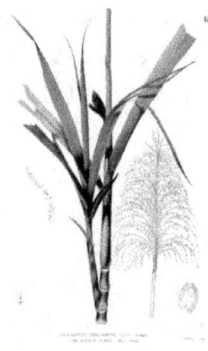

**Saccharumofficinarum** (Sugar Cane, Wax) Source of Policosanol

Policosanol, is an antilipemic agent that includes mixtures of aliphatic primary alcohols extracted from CeraeSaccharumOfficinarum (sugarcane wax) and is used in more than 25 countries to lower LDL cholesterol (Chen et al., 2005). The main components of sugarcane wax are octacosanol (62.9%), triacontanol (12.6%), and hexacosanol (6.2%) [Aneiros et al., 1993; Gouni-Berthold & Berthold, 2002].

Systematic review and meta-analysis of 29 randomized controlled trials evaluating the efficacy for policosanol 12 mg/day (range 5-40 mg/day [1528 patients-hypercholesterolemic/hyperlipidemic]) showed a reduction in LDL cholesterol, total cholesterol, triglyceride levels and an increase in HDL cholesterol (Chen et al., 2005).

Two studies demonstrated positive results using policosanol for patients with intermittent claudication.

Policosanol treatment decreased symptoms of claudication such as pain while exercising, intermittent pain, and lower extremity symptoms of coldness and pain (Castaño et al., 1999; Castaño et al., 2001c).

~~~~

Images by:
1. *Vitisvinifera* (Grape Berry, Seed: *Nikada (Living without Lupus)*
2. *Camellia sinensis* (Green Tea, Leaf): *Hortus Camdenensis,* © 2010–2012 by Colin Mills
3. *Vacciniummyrtillus* (Bilberry, Berry):  Vector Images
4. *Curcuma longa* (Turmeric,  Rhizome): Saai Anandhaa Exports
5. *Monascuspurpureus- Oryza* (Red Yeast Rice, Extract): "Oryza sativa at Kadavoor" © 2009 Jeevan Jose, Kerala
6. Saccharumofficinarum (Sugar Cane, Wax): Franz Eugen Köhler
7. *Pinus pinaster* (Maritime Pine, Bark): Scientific Illustration/BioDiv/Library - Flickr

# REFERENCES

*Detoxification: Powerful, Healthy, Healing*

*Cholesterol Facts and Fantasies*, Health Science Series #2 by Judith A. Deceive, BS, CAC

*Fats and Oils&Fats that Heal: Fats that Kill* by Udo Erasmus Alive Press, Vancouver BC (Two of the most thorough and valuable books)

*The Facts about Fats* by John Finnegan, an Elysian Arts book

*Coronaries, Cholesterol, Chlorine* by Dr. Joseph M. Price, a Pyramid book

Miscellaneous articles by Dr. Royal Lee and Dr. Richard Murray

ASSMANN G ET AL. (1996): High-density lipoprotein cholesterol as a predictor of coronary heart risk disease: the PROCAM experience and pathophysiological implications for reverse cholesterol transport. Atherosclerosis 124 (suppl 6): S11-S20

ATP III (2002): Third report of the National Cholesterol Education Program (NCEP) expert panel on detection, evaluation and treatment of high blood cholesterol in adults (Adult Treatment Panel III). Circulation 106: 3143 -3421

BERGE KE ET AL. (2000): Accumulation in dietary cholesterol in sitosterolemia caused by mutations in adjacent ABC transporters. Science 290: 1771-1775

BERGER A ET AL. (2004): Plant sterols: factors affecting their efficacy and safety as functional food ingredients. Lipids Health Dis 3:5

BROWN L ET AL. (1999): Cholesterol-lowering effects of dietary fiber: a meta-analysis; Am J ClinNutr 69: 30-42

CHENG TO (2006): Effects of fast food, rising blood pressure and increasing serum cholesterol on cardiovascular disease in China. Am J Cardiol 97(11): 1676-1678

COLMAN J (2005): Why our arteries become clogged with age. Life Extension Magazine Oct 2005

DANIELSEN EM ET AL. (1991): Morphological and functional changes in the enterocyte induced by fructose. Biochem J 280: 483-490

DAVIDSON MH (2005A): Lipoprotein metabolism and the pathogenesis of atherosclerosis. The mobile lipid clinic – a companion guide, pp 45-57

# ABOUT THE AUTHOR

Dr. Elvis Ali is highly respected for his work in Naturopathic Medicine. Dr. Elvis, as he is affectionately known, has been in private practice for over 30 years, specializing in Chinese and sports medicine and nutrition. With impressive credentials - Bachelor of Science, majoring in Biology, Licensed Acupuncturist, Doctorate in Naturopathic Medicine; Mind/Body Medicine at Harvard Medical School, Diploma in Homeopathic Medicine - he lectures internationally, has written several books and appeared on radio and television shows. His passion lies in empowering people by educating them on complementary health and wellness, and non-intrusive options.